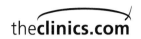

PSYCHIATRIC CLINICS
OF NORTH AMERICA

New Developments
in Depression Research

GUEST EDITORS
Dan V. Iosifescu, MD, MSc
and
Andrew A. Nierenberg, MD

March 2007 • Volume 30 • Number 1

SAUNDERS

An Imprint of Elsevier, Inc.
PHILADELPHIA   LONDON   TORONTO   MONTREAL   SYDNEY   TOKYO

W.B. SAUNDERS COMPANY
A Division of Elsevier Inc.

1600 John F. Kennedy Boulevard • Suite 1800 • Philadelphia, PA 19103-2899

http://www.theclinics.com

PSYCHIATRIC CLINICS OF NORTH AMERICA   Volume 30, Number 1
March 2007   ISSN 0193-953X
Editor: Sarah E. Barth   ISBN-13: 978-1-4160-4361-4
                                              ISBN-10: 1-4160-4361-6

Reprints. For copies of 100 or more, of articles in this publication, please contact the Commercial Reprints Department, Elsevier Inc., 360 Park Avenue South, New York, New York 10010-1710. Tel.: (212) 633-3813, Fax: (212) 462-1935, e-mail: reprints@elsevier.com.

The ideas and opinions expressed in *Psychiatric Clinics of North America* do not necessarily reflect those of the Publisher. The Publisher does not assume any responsibility for any injury and/or damage to persons or property arising out of or related to any use of the material contained in this periodical. The reader is advised to check the appropriate medical literature and the product information currently provided by the manufacturer of each drug to be administered, to verify the dosage, the method and duration of administration, or contraindications. It is the responsibility of the treating physician or other health care professional, relying on independent experience and knowledge of the patient, to determine drug dosages and the best treatment for the patient. Mention of any product in this issue should not be construed as endorsement by the contributors, editors, or the Publisher of the product or manufacturers' claims.

Psychiatric Clinics of North America (ISSN 0193-953X) is published quarterly by Elsevier Inc., 360 Park Avenue South, New York, NY 10010-1710. Months of issue are March, June, September, and December. Business and Editorial Offices: 1600 John F. Kennedy Blvd., Suite 1800, Philadelphia, PA 19103-2899. Customer Service Office: 6277 Sea Harbor Drive, Orlando, FL 32887-4800 Periodicals postage paid at New York, NY and additional mailing offices. Subscription prices are $194.00 per year (US individuals), $329.00 per year (US institutions), $97.00 per year (US students/residents), $232.00 per year (Canadian individuals), $400.00 per year (Canadian Institutions), $270.00 per year (foreign individuals), $400.00 per year (foreign institutions), and $135.00 per year (international & Canadian students/residents). Foreign air speed delivery is included in all *Clinics'* subscription prices. All prices are subject to change without notice. **POSTMASTER:** Send address changes to *Psychiatric Clinics of North America*, Elsevier Periodicals Customer Service, 6277 Sea Harbor Drive, Orlando, FL 32887-4800. Customer Service: 1-800-654-2452 (US). From outside of the US, call 1-407-345-4000.

Psychiatric Clinics of North America is covered in *Index Medicus, Current Contents/Social and Behavioral Sciences, Social Science Citation Index, Embase/Excerpta Medica,* and PsycINFO.

Printed in the United States of America.

New Developments in Depression Research

GUEST EDITORS

DAN V. IOSIFESCU, MD, MSc, Director of Neurophysiology Studies, Depression Clinical and Research Program; and Assistant Professor of Psychiatry, Massachusetts General Hospital, Harvard Medical School, Boston, Massachusetts

ANDREW A. NIERENBERG, MD, Associate Director, Depression Clinical and Research Program; Medical Director, Bipolar Clinic and Research Program; and Associate Professor of Psychiatry, Massachusetts General Hospital, Harvard Medical School, Boston, Massachusetts

CONTRIBUTORS

IAN A. COOK, MD, Associate Professor, Laboratory of Brain, Behavior, and Pharmacology, Semel Institute for Neuroscience and Human Behavior at UCLA, Department of Psychiatry and Biobehavioral Sciences, David Geffen School of Medicine at UCLA, Los Angeles, California

DARIN D. DOUGHERTY, MD, Director of Neurotherapeutics, Department of Psychiatry, Massachusetts General Hospital, Boston, Massachusetts

MAURIZIO FAVA, MD, Vice Chair, Department of Psychiatry; Depression Clinical and Research Program; and Professor of Psychiatry, Massachusetts General Hospital, Harvard Medical School, Boston, Massachusetts

GREG FELDMAN, PhD, Assistant Professor, Simmons College Department of Psychology; and Clinical and Research Fellow, Depression Clinical and Research Program, Department of Psychiatry, Massachusetts General Hospital, Boston, Massachusetts

AIMEE M. HUNTER, PhD, Assistant Research Psychologist, Laboratory of Brain, Behavior, and Pharmacology, Semel Institute for Neuroscience and Human Behavior at UCLA, Department of Psychiatry and Biobehavioral Sciences, David Geffen School of Medicine at UCLA, Los Angeles, California

DAN V. IOSIFESCU, MD, MSc, Director of Neurophysiology Studies, Depression Clinical and Research Program; and Assistant Professor of Psychiatry, Massachusetts General Hospital, Harvard Medical School, Boston, Massachusetts

JUDITH KATZ, BS, Depression Clinical and Research Program, Massachusetts General Hospital, Boston, Massachusetts

ANDREW F. LEUCHTER, MD, Professor, Laboratory of Brain, Behavior, and Pharmacology, Semel Institute for Neuroscience and Human Behavior at UCLA, Department of Psychiatry and Biobehavioral Sciences, David Geffen School of Medicine at UCLA, Los Angeles, California

DAVID MISCHOULON, MD, PhD, Director of Alternative Remedy Studies, Depression Clinical and Research Program; and Assistant Professor of Psychiatry, Massachusetts General Hospital, Harvard Medical School, Boston, Massachusetts

ANDREW A. NIERENBERG, MD, Associate Director, Depression Clinical and Research Program; Medical Director, Bipolar Clinic and Research Program; and Associate Professor of Psychiatry, Massachusetts General Hospital, Harvard Medical School, Boston, Massachusetts

MICHAEL J. OSTACHER, MD, MPH, Department of Psychiatry, Massachusetts General Hospital; and Department of Psychiatry, Harvard Medical School, Boston, Massachusetts

ROY H. PERLIS, MD, MSc, Director, Pharmacogenetics Research Unit, Depression and Bipolar Clinical and Research Programs and Center for Human Genetics Research, Massachusetts General Hospital, Boston, Massachusetts

SCOTT L. RAUCH, MD, President, Psychiatrist in Chief, Department of Psychiatry, McLean Hospital, Belmont, Massachusetts

RICHARD C. SHELTON, MD, James G. Blakemore Research Professor, Vice-Chair for Research, Department of Psychiatry; and Professor, Department of Pharmacology, Vanderbilt University Medical Center, Nashville, Tennessee

New Developments in Depression Research

The molecular neurobiology of depression begins with the concept that depressive disorders represent a family of related but distinct conditions. Different points of vulnerability in the brain may predispose a person to depressive disorders. Unraveling these complex causes may lead to novel treatments that can be used in a targeted fashion.

Major depressive disorder is a frequent, serious disorder that usually responds partially to treatment and leaves many patients with treatment resistance. This article reviews and critically evaluates the evidence for the management of treatment-resistant depression and examines pharmacologic approaches to alleviate the suffering of patients who benefit insufficiently from initial treatment.

Until recently, few treatments for major depression other than pharmacotherapy, psychotherapy, and electroconvulsive therapy have been available. This article reviews recent data from the field of somatic therapies for treatment-resistant depression. Examples of neurotherapeutic interventions for major depression include ablative limbic system surgeries (eg, anterior cingulotomy and subcaudate tractotomy), vagus nerve stimulation, transcranial magnetic stimulation, and deep brain stimulation. The article briefly discusses the role of each of these neurotherapeutic interventions in treating depression. It concludes with thoughts on the future potential of neurotherapeutic interventions in the treatment of depression.

Cognitive-behavioral therapy (CBT) is a nonpharmacologic strategy for depression treatment that has received considerable empirical support. This article provides an overview of the history and core techniques of CBT and discusses recently developed techniques and augmentations to CBT for depression. It reviews empirical studies comparing the relative efficacy of CBT and antidepressant medication as well as their combination. Studies highlighting the relapse-prevention properties of CBT are reviewed also. The article concludes with a discussion of practical recommendations for integrating CBT into a depression treatment plan.

The popularity of natural or "alternative" remedies to treat medical and psychiatric disorders has accelerated dramatically over the past decade, in the United States and worldwide. This article reviews the evidence for clinical efficacy, active ingredients, mechanisms of action, recommended dosages, and toxicities of the three best-studied putative natural antidepressants, St. John's Wort (hypericum), S-adenosyl methionine, and the omega-3 fatty acids eicosapentaenoic acid and docosahexaenoic acid. Despite growing evidence for efficacy and safety, more comprehensive studies are required before these remedies can be recommended as safe and effective alternatives or adjuncts to conventional psychotropic agents.

Major depressive disorder often co-occurs with substance use disorders, especially alcohol use disorders, and the course of each of these problems seems be complicated by the other. Diagnosing and treating these patients is challenging. A significant difficulty for clinicians is deciding whether to treat a mood episode in a patient who has current substance use or a substance use disorder, and what is the optimal treatment for that patient. This article discusses the prevalence of depressive and substance use disorder, the course of illness of comorbid depression and substance use disorders, and treatment response.

This article assesses the course of depressive disorders in persons who have comorbid medical illness. The article reviews a series of randomized, controlled studies of antidepressant treatment in subjects who have major depressive disorder (MDD) and selected medical illnesses. It also reviews a series of studies that compare the outcome of antidepressant treatment in subjects who have MDD with and without comorbid medical illness. It reviews hypotheses on the mechanism of the interaction between medical illness and clinical response in MDD. It concludes with clinical strategies recommended in depressed subjects who have medical comorbidity.

The ultimate goal of psychiatric research in major depressive disorder, including postmortem and neuroimaging studies, is better diagnosis and treatment of afflicted individuals. A growing number of neuroimaging studies have focused on correlates of treatment response. This article reviews findings from psychiatric research involving subjects who have major depression. It then discusses general issues involved in conducting neuroimaging studies that seek to identify correlates of treatment response. It concludes with a review of neuroimaging studies of treatment response in depression and integrates these findings into current models regarding the pathophysiology of major depression.

Quantitative electroencephalography (QEEG) has growing promise as an indicator of antidepressant treatment outcomes and as a tool that may become widespread in the clinical treatment of depression. Work across imaging modalities has shown that neurophysiologic function of the frontal brain region before treatment and early changes in frontal function after beginning antidepressant treatment are related to clinical outcomes later during treatment. Newer QEEG measurements are focusing on aspects of the electroencephalograph that are linked closely to cerebral perfusion and metabolism. QEEG biomarkers may become practical tools that can guide treatment for the individual patient.

FORTHCOMING ISSUES

June 2007
Clinical Interviewing
Shawn C. Shea, MD,
Guest Editor

September 2007
Schizophrenia
Erick L. Messias, MD, MPH, PhD and
Peter F. Buckley, MD,
Guest Editors

December 2007
Consultation – Liaison Psychiatry
James L. Levenson, MD, David F. Gitlin, MD, and
Cathy Crone, MD,
Guest Editors

RECENT ISSUES

December 2006
The Sleep-Psychiatry Interface
Karl Doghramji, MD,
Guest Editor

September 2006
Forensic Psychiatry
Charles L. Scott, MD,
Guest Editor

June 2006
Obsessive-Compulsive Spectrum Disorders
Dan J. Stein, MD, PhD,
Guest Editor

THE CLINICS ARE NOW AVAILABLE ONLINE!

Access your subscription at:
http://www.theclinics.com

Preface

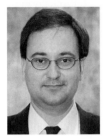
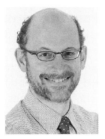

Dan V. Iosifescu, MD, MSc
Andrew A. Nierenberg, MD

Guest Editors

Major depressive disorder (MDD) challenges clinicians because it is common (with a 12-month prevalence of 7% [1] and lifetime prevalence of 20% [2]) and severe (more than 80% of patients have moderate to severe depression [1]) and because current treatments bring to acute and sustained remission only a minority of patients [3]. In the absence of useful clinical or biological predictors of response, clinicians have a limited basis to match treatments to patients, and researchers have limited targets to develop new treatments.

Most studies of interventions for MDD have focused on the short-term efficacy of antidepressants in relatively selected populations. In contrast, the Sequenced Treatment Alternatives To Relieve Depression (STAR*D) study, published in 2006, provides important longitudinal information about the real-world efficacy of currently used antidepressants as a first treatment and for those who have treatment-resistant depression (TRD). Other important developments in the treatment of TRD pertain to novel somatic treatments (including vagus nerve stimulation, recently approved by the Food and Drug Administration) and focused psychotherapies. Natural or alternative remedies also are growing in popularity. Recent studies have expanded the knowledge of real-world patients who have MDD by focusing on medical and psychiatric comorbidity, because such comorbid conditions can contribute to disease burden and can have a negative effect on treatment outcome.

One of the most promising developments in depression research is early data on biological markers of treatment outcome. Researchers have studied specific brain parameters measured by functional neuroimaging (functional MRI or

0193-953X/07/$ – see front matter
doi:10.1016/j.psc.2007.01.002

positron-emission tomography), electrophysiology (quantitative electroencepha-lography), or genetic tools to predict clinical outcomes of treatment with antide-pressants. Although most of these results are preliminary, and none of these biological markers has yet been sufficiently validated to warrant application in clinical practice, the development of these prognostic markers during the next de-cade looks promising. Such biological markers of treatment outcome could guide clinicians' selection of antidepressant agents in newly diagnosed patients and in those who have TRD. Researchers could also use such biomarkers to screen novel pharmacologic compounds assumed to have antidepressant efficacy.

This issue of *The Psychiatric Clinics of North America* aims to provide a clinically focused perspective to these recent developments in the rapidly expanding field of basic and clinical research in MDD. It begins with a review of the molecular neurobiology of depression. This review in turn focuses the discussion in the next several articles on treatment strategies for TRD (including pharmacologic agents, somatic treatments, psychotherapies, and alternative remedies). Two articles are dedicated to the important comorbidities of depression with alco-hol-misuse disorders and with medical illnesses. Articles then evaluate potential biologic markers of treatment outcome (defined by neuroimaging, electroen-cephalography, and genetic studies).

We are extraordinarily grateful for the scholarly contributions of all the au-thors, whose breadth of knowledge made possible the large scope of this issue. We hope these contributions will have a direct impact on your clinical practice and also prepare you for soon-to-arrive new developments in diagnostic and therapeutic tools.

Dan V. Iosifescu, MD, MSc
Massachusetts General Hospital
Harvard Medical School
50 Staniford Street, Suite 401
Boston, MA 02114, USA

E-mail address: diosifescu@partners.org

Andrew A. Nierenberg, MD
Massachusetts General Hospital
Harvard Medical School
50 Staniford Street, Suite 580
Boston, MA 02114, USA

E-mail address: aanierenberg@partners.org

References

[1] Kessler RC, Chiu WT, Demler O, et al. Prevalence, severity, and comorbidity of 12-month DSM-IV disorders in the National Comorbidity Survey Replication. Arch Gen Psychiatry 2005;62:617–27.

[2] Kessler RC, Berglund P, Demler O, et al. Lifetime prevalence and age-of-onset distributions of DSM-IV disorders in the National Comorbidity Survey Replication. Arch Gen Psychiatry 2005;62(6):593–602.

[3] Rush AJ, Kraemer HC, Sackeim HA, et al. Report by the ACNP Task Force on Response and Remission in Major Depressive Disorder. Neuropsychopharmacology 2006;31(9):1841–53.

The Molecular Neurobiology of Depression

Richard C. Shelton, MD[a,b,*]

[a]Department of Psychiatry, Vanderbilt University Medical Center, 1500 21st Avenue, South, Suite 2200, Nashville, TN 37212, USA
[b]Department of Pharmacology, Vanderbilt University Medical Center, 1500 21st Avenue, South, Suite 2200, Nashville, TN 37212, USA

Unipolar depressive disorders encompass a range of features that strongly suggest a neurobiologic substrate. These features include symptoms such as include sleep and appetite disturbances (both increases and decreases), loss of interest and pleasure, negative rumination, fatigue, and poor concentration and also apparent abnormalities of the hypothalamic-pituitary-adrenal (HPA) axis [1] or of neuroplasticity [2]. Moreover, depression seems to have genetic antecedents, also suggesting a biologic contribution to its origin [3]. The exact pathophysiology, however, has been largely unknown until the last decade or so.

Depression clearly is not one entity but includes a range of causes that involve genetic contributors along with early and later stress [2,4]. Therefore, the depressive spectrum includes conditions related to early traumatic events (typically with early onset of depression) through episodes in the absence of early trauma that may or may not be precipitated by an acute stressor. The heterogeneous nature of the condition must be taken into account in any search for a biologic substrate.

Unfortunately, that caveat usually is not observed. In fact, most studies simply take unselected groups of "depressed" and "control" subjects for comparison. This selection is likely to contribute to type II error, because a particular biologic finding may be applicable only to a subset of depressed patients. To illustrate this point, consider a study from the author's research laboratory at Vanderbilt University (Fig. 1) [5]. In this study, protein kinase A (PKA) activity was determined in fibroblasts in culture from a group of depressed patients and controls. Panel A of Fig. 1 shows the total group of depressed patients compared with normal controls. Clearly, some patients have reduced activity.

Supported in part by NIMH grants MH073630, MH01741, and MH52339.

*Department of Pharmacology, Vanderbilt University Medical Center, 1500 21st Avenue, South, Suite 2200, Nashville, TN 37212. E-mail address: richard.shelton@vanderbilt.edu

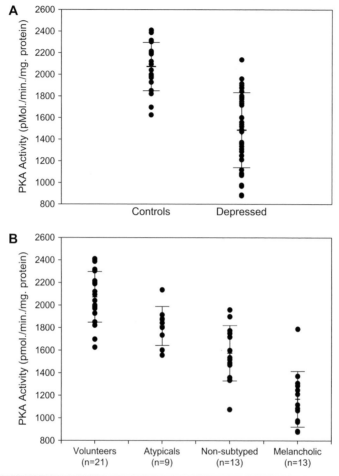

Fig. 1. Protein kinase A activity in depressed patients and normal controls. (*A*) Activity in the total group, depressed and controls. (*B*) Activity in depressive subtypes and controls. PKA, protein kinase A. (*Data from:* Shelton RC, Manier DH, Peterson CS, et al. Cyclic AMP-dependent protein kinase in subtypes of major depression and normal volunteers. Int J Neuro-psychopharmacol 1999;2(3):187–92.)

There is considerable overlap between the depressed and control populations, however. A different picture emerges when the depressed population is broken down by subtype. All the cells from patients who have atypical features fall within the control range. All but one melancholic patient were outside the range; the subjects not subtyped as melancholic or atypical fall between. This figure indicates that a particular finding, low PKA activity, is characteristic of only one subset of depressed patients. Similar data in human postmortem brain indicate that the reduced PKA activity may be associated with death by suicide [6,7]. Together, these results indicate that there will not be a single, unitary set of biologic substrates that explain the full range of depressive disorders. Further, all contributors, such as genetic antecedents, early trauma, and recent stress, confer their own, perhaps unique, mechanisms of etiology

THE ROLE OF STRESS

That life stressors contribute in some fashion to depression is almost a truism and essentially is an extension of what occurs normally. That is, adverse events confer negative mood states in normal persons. The search for physiologic underpinnings, therefore, can be thought of as an extrapolation (and, hence, dysregulation) of normal responses in many circumstances [8]; this concept is discussed in greater detail later. The work of Kendler and colleagues [9,10] suggests that the both early and recent adversity contribute significantly to the potential for a depressive episode [9,10]. Moreover, early adverse events, particularly abuse, seem to confer heightened risk [9,11–14], an issue that reappears later in the discussion of cellular pathology.

The interplay of genetics and environment is highly complex, and research in this area is in its infancy. Caspi and colleagues [15] have demonstrated a causal interaction between a specific polymorphic variant of the serotonin transporter (5HT-T), early and late adversity, and the occurrence of depression. This group investigated the contribution of a common and functional polymorphism of the promoter region of the 5HT-T gene (*5HTTLPR*). 5HT-T is the principal modular of synaptic serotonin (5HT) activity and is blocked by serotonin-selective reuptake inhibitors. This study evaluated 847 people followed over the course of 2 decades. The results suggested an interaction between the functional, so-called "short" (s) variant of *5HTTLPR* with both early and late adversity. For example, stressful events were tabulated for the period between ages 21 and 26 years. There was no relationship between the s variant and the occurrence of depression in participants who reported no major stressors during this period. The occurrence of stressors, however, conferred increased risk, primarily in persons carrying the s allele. Moreover, there was an environmental stress-dose effect; that is, more stressful events produced higher risk. There also was a gene-dose effect in which the short-short (ss) carriers had the highest risk, the long-long (ll) carriers had the lowest, with the ls carriers falling in between. There also was a relationship between early traumas and risk for depression that was modulated by genotype. Specifically, persons who had no history of early maltreatment did not show any association between transporter alleles and depression. In those who did have early maltreatment, the risk segregated according to allelic status, with the ss carriers having the highest risk. Again, there was both a stress-dose and gene-dose effect. These results were confirmed in a recent study with a new cohort [16]. These results suggest a strong interaction between genetic diathesis (and, hence, biologic substrate) and both early and recent stressors. Although this interaction is a complicating element, it opens particular avenues of investigation.

STRESS AND THE HYPOTHALAMIC-PITUITARY-ADRENAL AXIS DYSFUNCTION: RISK FOR DEPRESSION

Abnormalities of the HPA axis in depressed patients are well described [1]. Overt dysregulation is found only in a subset of depressed patients, however. As articulated by Nemeroff and colleagues [17,18], depression and early trauma converge at the level of HPA-axis regulation. Adversity that occurs early in life and is severe and prolonged seems to contribute significantly both to subsequent risk for anxiety and depressive disorders and to HPA dysfunction. Traumas such as physical or sexual abuse or the loss of a parent that occur during critical periods of development result in a permanent alteration of stress reactivity in the central nervous system. Actually, from a teleologic perspective, the maintenance of an activated stress response system following chronic or severe stress makes adaptive sense, in that high threat intensity would result in a persistently elevated "alert" status.

Persistent enhancement of stress reactivity could explain the findings of heightened HPA-axis activity, including elevated peripheral cortisol [1,19,20] and central corticotrophin-releasing hormone [21,22], in some depressed patients. The interplay of genetic predisposition and early adversity then would lead to a vulnerable phenotype. Moreover, this interplay is likely to result in heightened stress reactivity by at least two mechanisms. The first would be the biologic diathesis. The second would be a pattern of maladaptive responses to stressors. For example, withdrawal from a stressor would be highly adaptive in the case of early abuse. That same behavior manifested in adult life would be equally maladaptive. These factors, then, would combine to elevate risk for depression.

Alternatively, the fact that not all depressed persons have been abused in childhood would explain why only a subset shows HPA activation. The etiologic pathways and the subcellular dysfunction associated with it could differ in depressed persons who do not have a history of early adversity.

INTRACELLULAR SIGNAL TRANSDUCTION

A number of studies implicate intracellular signal transduction in the pathophysiology of depression. One key set of mechanisms involves phosphorylation enzymes, including PKA and protein kinase C (PKC) (Fig. 2). The binding of a transmitter with a G-protein–linked receptor activates the coupling of G-proteins (Gs and Gq) with second-messenger enzymes such adelylate cyclase or phospholipase C. These enzymes in turn catalyze the formation of the second messengers cyclic AMP and diacylglycerol. These second messengers then bind to PKA and PKC, respectively, facilitating phosphorylation by these enzymes [23].

Protein kinases are critical elements of stimulus–response coupling [24]. One critical effect is the subsequent phosphorylation of the transcription factor cyclic AMP response element binding protein (CREB). CREB phosphorylation is linked to both norepinephrine- and 5-HT–linked cascades and may represent a common target of action of more noradrenergic and serotonergic

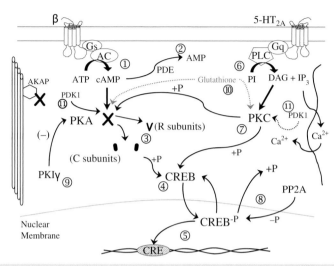

Fig. 2. Cell surface receptors, such as norepinephrine β receptors, are coupled to stimulatory G (Gs) proteins. (1) On transmitter binding, Gs activates adenylate cyclase (AC), catalyzing the formation of cyclic AMP from ATP. (2) Cyclic AMP is degraded to AMP by phosphodiesterases (PDE), which inactivate the cyclic AMP signal. (3) Cyclic AMP binds to the regulator subunits (R) of protein kinase A (PKA), resulting in a conformational change and the release of two catalytic subunits (C). (4) The C subunits then are capable of phosphorylating serine and threonine residues on target polypeptides. One such protein is cyclic AMP response element binding protein (CREB), a transcriptional factor. (5) Phosphorylation of CREB results in translocation of CREB-P to the nucleus and subsequent binding to CRE-containing gene-promoter regions activating expression. (6) A parallel pathway, exemplified by the 5-HT$_{2A}$ transductional cascade, couples to Gq (another stimulatory G protein), activating phospholipase C (PLC) catalyzing the conversion of phosphatidylinositol (PI) to diacylglycerol (DAG) and inositol triphosphate (IP$_3$). (7) IP$_3$ mobilizes Ca^{2+} release from intracellular stores. DAG binds to protein kinase C (PKC) resulting in phosphorylation of target proteins; these include both CREB and PKA. (8) The phosphorylation of PKA regulates the activity of the enzyme. Phosphorylated substrates are subsequently dephosphorylated by protein phosphatase 2A. (9) On dephosphorylation, CREB returns to the cytosol. Another regulator of PKA activity is protein kinase inhibitor (PKI); in the case of fibroblasts, this is the PKIγ isoform. (10) Both PKA and PKC can be glutathionylated, protecting them from oxidative degradation. The activation loops of both enzymes are phosphorylated by phosphoinositide dependent kinase 1 (PDK1).

antidepressants [24]. Phosphorylated CREB binds to cyclic AMP response element in the promoter region of genes, which regulates gene expression [25]. This binding represents an integrative set of mechanisms in which antidepressants acting through either norepinephrine or 5-HT can target a common set of genes and their respective protein products.

A variety of research has implicated deficiencies in PKA and PKC in a subset of depressives [26]. For example, the research group at Vanderbilt University has shown that, relative to normal controls, certain depressed patients have deficient PKA and PKC protein levels [27,28], lower binding of cyclic AMP to PKA [29], reduced phosphorylation of CREB [29], and altered gene-expression patterns [30]. These findings also have been shown in both peripheral and post-mortem brain tissues by other groups [6,7,31–39]. This decrease in the activity of these two key enzymes would be expected to alter the expression of genes that contain cyclic AMP response element in their promoters; these would include key proteins that regulate the stress response in brain, including brain-derived neurotrophic factor (BDNF) [40–42], the BDNF receptor trk-b [43], and glucocorticoid receptor (GR) [44]. Moreover, GR functions as a transcriptional factor and regulates the expression of other genes, specifically exerting an inhibitory effect on corticotrophin-releasing hormone [45]. Hence, reduced activity of these key enzymes could enhance stress reactivity through altered regulation of the expression of specific genes. Important elements of stress regulation could be vulnerable under demand conditions. In fact, the knockout of PKA and PKC protein isoforms in mice has demonstrated a variety of cellular effects [46,47], most particularly hippocampal neuroplasticity [46,48], which has been implicated in depression [49].

MECHANISMS FOR ALTERED PROTEIN ACTIVITY

Although the evidence for altered kinase activity seems sound, the exact mechanisms for inducing these effects are unknown. One possible avenue is through protein oxidation. The oxidation–reduction (redox) potential is altered by reactive oxygen species (ROS), which are formed by a variety of factors, including inflammatory cytokines [50]. Altered redox potential has been shown to affect the activity of kinases [50]. Glutathione, an intracellular antioxidant, is involved in the protection of proteins against oxidative stress [50–52] by binding to redox-sensitive amino acids (particularly cysteine). Recently, glutathionylation has been described as an important regulator of PKA degradation [53] and could be involved in the availability of PKA proteins.

As noted, proinflammatory cytokines are involved in the genesis of ROS and thereby affect oxidation and, hence, degradation of proteins. Altered cytokine activity is well-described in depression [54], and antidepressant drugs have been shown to regulate the expression of specific cytokines, in particular by inhibiting proinflammatory cytokines that are involved in enhancing ROS [55]. Curiously, this activity seems to be mediated through kinase-related pathways. Maes and colleagues [56] showed that the inhibitory effects of fluoxetine on tumor necrosis factor alpha are mediated, in part, by PKA. This inhibition suggests an interactive system in which kinase-dependent pathways may modulate cytokine expression, and proinflammatory cytokines may affect kinase-dependent pathways through protein oxidation.

Another key element in regulation of stress responsivity is epigenetic regulation of gene expression. DNA does not exist in an unregulated, open fashion. DNA is associated with histone proteins that determine gene expression to a significant extent [57,58]. A number of protein-modification processes, including phosphorylation, acetylation, methylation, ubiquitination, and ribosylation, can influence these proteins as they do other protein elements in cells [58,59]. Furthermore, direct methylation of DNA sequences, particularly promoter regions, exerts major influences on activity. Methylation, a key determinant of DNA expression, occurs on cytosines of the dinucleotide cytosine phosphate guanine (CpG) through DNA methyltransferases [58,59]. These mechanisms, termed "epigenetic regulation," represent inducible and potentially reversible phenomena that can be modified by environmental factors. These effects may, then, mediate gene–environment interactions and determine both short- and longer-term responses to environmental cues [58,59].

This concept was tested recently in an elegant set of experiments from the laboratory of Dr. Michael Meaney [60–66]. Rat mothers periodically engage in licking and grooming (LG) and arched-back nursing (ABN) of their pups. They show a range of such responses, however, with some mothers showing high and others low levels of LG-ABN behaviors. Lowlevel LG-ABN behavior in the mothers was associated with a marked elevation in methylation of exon 1_7 of the GR promoter region in the pups when compared with pups who received high levels of LG-ABN behavior, an effect that persisted into adult life. The cross-fostering of pups reversed this pattern, indicating that maternal behavior was the mediator. This increased promoter methylation resulted in decreased GR expression in brain and a heightened corticosterone response to stress. These data indicate a causal relationship between maternal behavior and subsequent stress reactivity that is mediated by methylation of a specific gene.

SUMMARY

Depression is a condition with a complex biologic pattern of etiology. Environmental stressors modulate subsequent vulnerability to depression. In particular, early adversity seems to induce heightened reactivity to stress through several possible mechanisms, both biologic and psychologic. This increased reactivity results in an enhancement of biologic stress-response mechanisms, especially the HPA axis. Regulators of this system, particularly signal transduction pathways involving PKA and PKC, may be important in the regulation of key genes in this system including genes for GR, BDNF, and trk-b. This system potentially is vulnerable to ROS and therefore, indirectly, to the effects of cytokines. Finally, some of these effects may be controlled by chemical modification of DNA, specifically, methylation of promoters or other gene regions. This modification is a mechanism by which long-term biologic change can be induced by environmental stressors.

The brain is homeostatic, and it is possible that alterations at multiple points in this system may induce dysregulation and, as a result, vulnerability to stress. Therefore, a person may be vulnerable to depression, which may be a final common "pathway" for this family of conditions. Individuals may vary considerably with regard to the locus of the problem, however. For example, functional variants in a set of genes might predispose some people to depression; others may have epigenetic imprinting; and yet different causes may be at work in others. Although this mix is complicated, it can be unraveled. Doing so could lead to the development of novel interventions that could target specific points of vulnerability, allowing an improved matching of patient to treatment based on differential abnormalities at the cellular level.

References

[1] Gillespie CF, Nemeroff CB. Hypercortisolemia and depression. Psychosom Med 2005;67(Suppl 1):S26–8.

[2] Hayley S, Poulter MO, Merali Z, et al. The pathogenesis of clinical depression: stressor- and cytokine-induced alterations of neuroplasticity. Neuroscience 2005;135(3):659–78.

[3] Kendler KS, Davis CG, Kessler RC. The familial aggregation of common psychiatric and substance use disorders in the National Comorbidity Survey: a family history study. Br J Psychiatry 1997;170:541–8.

[4] Kendler KS, Kessler RC, Walters EE, et al. Stressful life events, genetic liability, and onset of an episode of major depression in women. Am J Psychiatry 1995;153:833–42.

[5] Shelton RC, Manier DH, Peterson CS, et al. Cyclic AMP-dependent protein kinase in subtypes of major depression and normal volunteers. Int J Neuropsychopharmacol 1999; 2(3):187–92.

[6] Dwivedi Y, Conley RR, Roberts RC, et al. [(3)H]cAMP binding sites and protein kinase a activity in the prefrontal cortex of suicide victims. Am J Psychiatry 2002;159(1):66–73.

[7] Dwivedi Y, Rizavi HS, Shukla PK, et al. Protein kinase A in postmortem brain of depressed suicide victims: altered expression of specific regulatory and catalytic subunits. Biol Psychiatry 2004;55(3):234–43.

[8] Shelton RC. Intracellular mechanisms of antidepressant drug action. Harv Rev Psychiatry 2000;8(4):161–74.

[9] Kendler KS, Gardner CO, Prescott CA. Toward a comprehensive developmental model for major depression in women. Am J Psychiatry 2002;159(7):1133–45.

[10] Kendler KS, Gardner CO, Prescott CA. Toward a comprehensive developmental model for major depression in men. Am J Psychiatry 2006;163(1):115–24.

[11] Kendler KS, Kuhn JW, Prescott CA. Childhood sexual abuse, stressful life events and risk for major depression in women. Psychol Med 2004;34(8):1475–82.

[12] Kendler KS, Sheth K, Gardner CO, et al. Childhood parental loss and risk for first-onset of major depression and alcohol dependence: the time-decay of risk and sex differences. Psychol Med 2002;32(7):1187–94.

[13] Kendler KS, Thornton LM, Gardner CO. Genetic risk, number of previous depressive episodes, and stressful life events in predicting onset of major depression. Am J Psychiatry 2001;158(4):582–6.

[14] Kendler KS, Thornton LM, Gardner CO. Stressful life events and previous episodes in the etiology of major depression in women: an evaluation of the "kindling" hypothesis. Am J Psychiatry 2000;157(8):1243–51.

[15] Caspi A, Sugden K, Moffitt TE, et al. Influence of life stress on depression: moderation by a polymorphism in the 5-HTT gene. Science 2003;301(5631):386–9.

[16] Kendler KS, Kuhn JW, Vittum J, et al. The interaction of stressful life events and a serotonin transporter polymorphism in the prediction of episodes of major depression: a replication. Arch Gen Psychiatry 2005;62(5):529–35.

[17] Heim C, Plotsky PM, Nemeroff CB. Importance of studying the contributions of early adverse experience to neurobiological findings in depression. Neuropsychopharmacology 2004; 29(4):641–8.

[18] Nemeroff CB. Neurobiological consequences of childhood trauma. J Clin Psychiatry 2004;65(Suppl 1):18–28.

[19] Wong M-L, Kling MA, Munson PJ. Pronounced and sustained central hypernoradrenergic function in mahor depression with melancholic features: relation to hypercortisolism and corticotrophin-releasing hormone. Proc Natl Acad Sci U S A 2000;97:325–30.

[20] Gold PW, Drevets WC, Charney DS. New insights into the role of cortisol and the glucocorticoid receptor in severe depression. Biol Psychiatry 2002;52(5):381–5.

[21] Heuser I, Bissette G, Dettling M, et al. Cerebrospinal fluid concentrations of corticotropin-releasing hormone, vasopressin, and somatostatin in depressed patients and healthy controls: response to amitriptyline treatment. Depress Anxiety 1998;8(2):71–9.

[22] Banki CM, Karmacsi L, Bissette G, et al. CSF corticotropin-releasing hormone and somatostatin in major depression: response to antidepressant treatment and relapse. Eur Neuropsychopharmacol 1992;2(2):107–13.

[23] Nestler EJ, Greengard P. Protein phosphorylation in the nervous system. New York: John Wiley & Sons; 1984.

[24] Hyman SE, Nestler EJ. Initiation and adaptation: a paradigm for understanding psychotropic drug action. Am J Psychiatry 1996;153(2):151–62.

[25] Yamamoto KK, Gonzalez GA, Biggs WH III, et al. Phosphorylation-induced binding and transcriptional efficacy of nuclear factor CREB. Nature 1988;334(6182):494–8.

[26] Pandey GN, Dwivedi Y. Focus on protein kinase A and protein kinase C, critical components of signal transduction system, in mood disorders and suicide. Int J Neuropsychopharmacol 2005;8:1–4.

[27] Akin D, Manier DH, Sanders-Bush E, et al. Decreased serotonin $5-HT_{2A}$ receptor-stimulated phosphoinositide signaling in fibroblasts from melancholic depressed patients. Neuropsychopharmacology 2004;29:2081–7.

[28] Akin D, Manier DH, Sanders-Bush E, et al. Signal transduction abnormalities in melancholic depression. Int J Neuropsychopharmacol 2005;8:5–16.

[29] Manier DH, Shelton RC, Ellis TC, et al. Human fibroblasts as a relevant model to study signal transduction in affective disorders. J Affect Disord 2000;61(1–2):51–8.

[30] Shelton RC, Liang S, Liang P, et al. Differential expression of pentraxin 3 in fibroblasts from patients with major depression. Neuropsychopharmacology 2004;29:126–32.

[31] Pandey GN, Dwivedi Y, Pandey SC, et al. Protein kinase C in the postmortem brain of teenage suicide victims. Neurosci Lett 1997;228(2):111–4.

[32] Pandey GN, Dwivedi Y, Kumari R, et al. Protein kinase C in platelets of depressed patients. Biol Psychiatry 1998;44:909–11.

[33] Pandey GN, Dwivedi Y, SridharaRao J, et al. Protein kinase C and phospholipase C activity and expression of their specific isozymes is decreased and expression of MARCKS is increased in platelets of bipolar but not in unipolar patients. Neuropsychopharmacology 2002;26(2):216–28.

[34] Dwivedi Y, Rao JS, Rizavi HS, et al. Abnormal expression and functional characteristics of cyclic adenosine monophosphate response element binding protein in postmortem brain of suicide subjects. Arch Gen Psychiatry 2003;60(3):273–82.

[35] Pandey GN, Dwivedi Y, Ren X, et al. Decreased protein expression and CRE–DNA binding activity of cyclic adenosine monophosphate response element binding protein in neutrophil of depressed patients. Presented at the annual meeting of the American College of Neuropsychopharmacology. San Juan, PR; December 7–11, 2003.

[36] Hrdina P, Faludi G, Li Q, et al. Growth-associated protein (GAP-43), its mRNA, and protein kinase C (PKC) isoenzymes in brain regions of depressed suicides. Mol Psychiatry 1998; 3(5):411–8.

[37] Coull MA, Lowther S, Katona CL, et al. Altered brain protein kinase C in depression: a postmortem study. Eur Neuropsychopharmacol 2000;10(4):283–8.

[38] Perez J, Tardito D, Racagni G, et al. Protein kinase A and Rap1 levels in platelets of untreated patients with major depression. Mol Psychiatry 2001;6(1):44–9.

[39] Perez J, Tardito D, Racagni G, et al. cAMP signaling pathway in depressed patients with psychotic features. Mol Psychiatry 2002;7(2):208–12.

[40] Shieh PB, Hu SC, Bobb K, et al. Identification of a signaling pathway involved in calcium regulation of BDNF expression. Neuron 1998;20(4):727–40.

[41] Meller R, Babity JM, Grahame-Smith DG. 5-HT2A receptor activation leads to increased BDNF mRNA expression in C6 glioma cells. NeuroMolecular Med 2002;1(3): 197–205.

[42] Karege F, Schwald M, El Kouaissi R. Drug-induced decrease of protein kinase a activity reveals alteration in BDNF expression of bipolar affective disorder. Neuropsychopharmacology 2004;29(4):805–12.
[43] Deogracias R, Espliguero G, Iglesias T, et al. Expression of the neurotrophin receptor trkB is regulated by the cAMP/CREB pathway in neurons. Mol Cell Neurosci 2004;26(3): 470–80.
[44] Barrett TJ, Vedeckis WV. Occupancy and composition of proteins bound to the AP-1 sites in the glucocorticoid receptor and c-jun promoters after glucocorticoid treatment and in different cell types. Recept Signal Transduct 1996;6(3–4):179–93.
[45] Malkoski SP, Dorin RI. Composite glucocorticoid regulation at a functionally defined negative glucocorticoid response element of the human corticotropin-releasing hormone gene. Mol Endocrinol 1999;13(10):1629–44.
[46] Qi M, Zhuo M, Skalhegg BS, et al. Impaired hippocampal plasticity in mice lacking the Cbeta1 catalytic subunit of cAMP-dependent protein kinase. Proc Natl Acad Sci U S A 1996; 93(4):1571–6.
[47] Dempsey EC, Newton AC, Mochly-Rosen D, et al. Protein kinase C isozymes and the regulation of diverse cell responses. Am J Physiol Lung Cell Mol Physiol 2000;279(3): L429–38.
[48] Nguyen PV, Woo NH. Regulation of hippocampal synaptic plasticity by cyclic AMP-dependent protein kinases. Prog Neurobiol 2003;71(6):401–37.
[49] Duman RS. Synaptic plasticity and mood disorders. Mol Psychiatry 2002;7(Suppl 1): S29–34.
[50] Adler V, Yin Z, Tew KD, et al. Role of redox potential and reactive oxygen species in stress signaling. Oncogene 1999;18(45):6104–11.
[51] Dickinson DA, Moellering DR, Iles KE, et al. Cytoprotection against oxidative stress and the regulation of glutathione synthesis. Biol Chem 2003;384(4):527–37.
[52] Dickinson DA, Forman HJ. Glutathione in defense and signaling: lessons from a small thiol. Ann N Y Acad Sci 2002;973:488–504.
[53] Humphries KM, Juliano C, Taylor SS. Regulation of cAMP-dependent protein kinase activity by glutathionylation. J Biol Chem 2002;277(45):43505–11.
[54] Licinio J, Wong ML. The role of inflammatory mediators in the biology of major depression: central nervous system cytokines modulate the biological substrate of depressive symptoms, regulate stress-responsive systems, and contribute to neurotoxicity and neuroprotection . [review] [92 refs]. Mol Psychiatry 1999;4(4):317–27.
[55] Maes M. The immunoregulatory effects of antidepressants. Hum Psychopharmacol 2001;16(1):95–103.
[56] Maes M, Kenis G, Kubera M, et al. The negative immunoregulatory effects of fluoxetine in relation to the cAMP-dependent PKA pathway. Int Immunopharmacol 2005;5(3):609–18.
[57] Jenuwein T, Allis CD. Translating the histone code. [See comment]. Science 2001; 293(5532):1074–80.
[58] Egger G, Liang G, Aparicio A, et al. Epigenetics in human disease and prospects for epigenetic therapy. Nature 2004;429:457–63.
[59] Jaenisch R, Bird A. Epigenetic regulation of gene expression: how the genome integrates intrinsic and environmental signals. [review] [186 refs]. Nat Genet 2003;33(Suppl):54.
[60] Champagne FA, Weaver IC, Diorio J, et al. Maternal care associated with methylation of the estrogen receptor-alpha1b promoter and estrogen receptor-alpha expression in the medial preoptic area of female offspring. Endocrinology 2006;147:2909–15.
[61] Weaver IC, Champagne FA, Brown SE, et al. Reversal of maternal programming of stress responses in adult offspring through methyl supplementation: altering epigenetic marking later in life. J Neurosci 2005;25:11045–54.
[62] Szyf M, Weaver IC, Champagne FA, et al. Maternal programming of steroid receptor expression and phenotype through DNA methylation in the rat. Front Neuroendocrinol 2005;26:139–62.

[63] Meaney MJ, Szyf M. Environmental programming of stress responses through DNA methyl-
     ation: life at the interface between a dynamic environment and a fixed genome. Dialogues
     Clin Neurosci 2005;7:103–23.
[64] Fish EW, Shahrokh D, Bagot R, et al. Epigenetic programming of stress responses through
     variations in maternal care. Ann N Y Acad Sci 2004;1036:167–80.
[65] Weaver IC, Cervoni N, Champagne FA, et al. Epigenetic programming by maternal behav-
     ior. Nat Neurosci 2004;7:847–54.
[66] Weaver IC, Szyf M, Meaney MJ. From maternal care to gene expression: DNA methylation
     and the maternal programming of stress responses. Endocr Res 2002;28:699.

A Critical Overview of the Pharmacologic Management of Treatment-Resistant Depression

Andrew A. Nierenberg, MD*, Judith Katz, BS, Maurizio Fava, MD

Depression Clinical and Research Program, Massachusetts General Hospital, 50 Staniford Street, Boston, MA 02114, USA

M ajor depressive disorder (MDD) has a lifetime prevalence of about 17% to 21%, with about twice as many women affected as men [1]. In any 12-month period, the prevalence of MDD is about 6.7%, with more than 80% of patients who have MDD experiencing moderate to severe depression [2]. Most patients do not receive timely treatment [3], even though the disorder disrupts functioning at work, home, and school [4]. The National Comorbidity Replication study showed that about 38% of those who experience a major depressive episode receive at least minimally adequate care in mental health specialty or general medical settings [5], leaving the majority of patients with inadequate treatment. For patients who do receive adequate pharmacotherapy, it is estimated from randomized, controlled trials of antidepressants that about 30% to 40% achieve full remission (absence or near absence of symptoms), leaving 60% to 70% who fail to reach remission [6]. About 10% to 15% have no response (at least a 50% improvement) [7]. Nonresponse is associated with disability and higher medical costs [8], and partial response and response without remission are associated with higher relapse and recurrence rates [9,10].

Thus MDD is a frequent, serious disorder that usually responds partially to treatment and leaves many patients with treatment resistance. This article reviews and critically evaluates the evidence for the management of treatment-resistant depression (TRD) and examines pharmacologic approaches to alleviate the suffering of patients who benefit insufficiently from initial treatment.

DIAGNOSTIC REASSESSMENT

Typically, the first step in the management of patients who have TRD involves a diagnostic reassessment. Errors of omission in the initial diagnosis of

*Corresponding author. Suite 580, 50 Staniford Street, Boston, MA 02114. E-mail address: anierenberg@partners.org (A.A. Nierenberg).

0193-953X/07/$ – see front matter
doi:10.1016/j.psc.2007.01.001

psychiatric comorbidity can have a negative impact on treatment outcome. One of the lessons learned from the National Comorbidity Replication study is that most patients who have MDD have comorbid conditions that, in turn, can contribute to disease burden and could prevent a full response to treatment [4]. For example, 57.5% of patients who have had MDD in the past 12 months also have had an anxiety disorder within the past 12 months, and about 9% have adult attention deficit hyperactivity disorder (ADHD) [11]. Although it would seem obvious that clinicians should treat patients' comorbid conditions to help achieve full remission, what is less obvious is how clinicians can identify and diagnose those comorbid conditions that appear in routine practice and avoid errors of omission. Instruments such as the Mini-International Neuropsychiatric Interview [12] or the structured clinical interview for the *Diagnostic and Statistic Manual of Mental Disorders*, edition 4 [13] are used routinely in research settings but are not used frequently in clinical settings. Perhaps clinicians need not conduct such extensive research evaluations on every patient at the outset of treatment but instead should provide a more systematic and comprehensive evaluation if a patient continues to feel depressed despite adequate treatment. Instruments such as the Psychiatric Diagnostic Screening Questionnaire could be considered [14].

ESTABLISHING TREATMENT GOALS

Remission of MDD (ie, full resolution of depressive symptoms) should be the ultimate goal of treatment [6]. Remission, in contrast to response (ie, a 50% reduction in baseline depressive symptoms), is associated with lower levels of disability and dysfunction [8] and a lower likelihood of relapse and recurrence [15]. Thus when adequately administered treatments fail to bring patients who have MDD to remission, those episodes can be classified as treatment resistant [16–18].

PHARMACOLOGIC OPTIONS

Pharmacologic options to manage TRD include augmentation, combination, and switching to another antidepressant. With the exception of the Sequenced Treatment Alternatives to Relieve Depression (STAR*D) project, most of the literature on pharmacologic options focuses on short-term efficacy. Few examine long-term efficacy. One includes a placebo-controlled substitution paradigm to assess the necessity for continuation treatment with an augmenting agent.

Augmentation

Augmentation can be defined as the use of a psychotropic agent that does not have an indication for depression to enhance the effect of an antidepressant. The theoretical rationale of augmentation is to obtain a different neurochemical effect by adding an agent affecting different neurotransmitter systems. Additionally, an augmentation agent can be used to broaden the therapeutic effect (eg, by adding an antianxiety agent to an antidepressant).

Among the most widely studied augmentation agents is lithium augmentation (>600 mg/d) of tricyclic antidepressants (TCAs), monoamine oxidase inhibitors (MAOIs), and selective serotonin reuptake inhibitors (SSRIs) [19].

Disadvantages of lithium augmentation include relatively low response rates in most recent studies [20–22], the risk of toxicity [23], and the need for blood monitoring. An advantage of lithium augmentation is the substantial body of data supporting its efficacy. The pooled odds ratio from nine studies of response during lithium augmentation compared with placebo is 3.31 (95% confidence interval [CI], 1.46–7.53) [19]. Even with these supporting data, less than 0.5% of depressed patients received lithium augmentation in a large pharmacoepidemiology study [24]. On balance, lithium augmentation can be considered a reasonable option, with the caveat that its efficacy may be rather limited with the newer generation of antidepressants.

Thyroid hormone augmentation T3 (25–50 µg/d) is another option that has received attention over the years [25]. L-triiodothyronine has been used in preference to and has been thought superior to thyroxine [26]. The disadvantages of thyroid augmentation are that all published controlled studies concern TCAs [25], and only uncontrolled studies pertain to SSRIs [27–29]. Of note, Iosifescu and colleagues found that brain energy metabolism increased among patients who responded to thyroid augmentation, whereas there was no change in brain energy metabolism in those who did not respond (D. Iosifescu, personal communication, 2006). Among the four randomized, double-blind studies, pooled effects were not significant (relative response, 1.53; 95% CI, 0.70–3.35; $P = .29$) [25]. The STAR*D study used an effectiveness design to compare lithium with thyroid augmentation in patients who had not reached remission with at least two prospective antidepressant trials [22]. Thyroid was given openly, but assessments were done either by assessors blind to treatment or by self report. Twenty-four percent of patients reached remission with thyroid, and there was a nonsignificantly greater improvement than with lithium augmentation.

In theory, buspirone, a 5-HT1A partial agonist (10–30 mg twice daily) used early in open augmentation trials of antidepressants [30], should augment SSRIs by blunting the negative feedback of increased synaptic serotonin effects on the presynaptic 5-HT1A receptor. The data are equivocal, however. The only two placebo-controlled studies showed buspirone was no better than placebo [31,32]. In one of the two negative studies, buspirone was better than placebo in severe depression [32]. The STAR*D study compared buspirone with bupropion and found that both helped about 30% of patients who had not reached remission [33]. One particular advantage of buspirone is that it may be helpful in SSRI-induced sexual dysfunction among women [34].

Pindolol, a beta-blocker and a 5-HT1A antagonist (2.5 mg three times daily), [35] initially was thought to have great potential because of its ability (similar to that of buspirone) to block the negative feedback of serotonin on presynaptic 5-HT1A receptors. Disadvantages from published studied are that the dose used may be too low, according to positron emission tomographic studies [36]; that no response was found in a group of 10 patients who had TRD [37]; and that no difference from placebo was found in two TRD studies [38,39]. In addition, one report suggested that pindolol may cause increased irritability [40]. An advantage of pindolol is that it has been shown to accelerate response to SSRIs in most, but not all, double-blind studies [41].

Dopaminergic agonists have been particularly interesting because they bring in a mechanism of action missing from antidepressants. Pergolide (0.25–2 mg/d) [42,43], amantadine (100–200 mg twice daily) [44], pramipexole (0.125–1 mg three times daily) [45,46], and ropinirole (0.5–1.75 mg twice daily) [47] have been found to be helpful in uncontrolled studies in patients who had MDD. Disadvantages include the side of effect of nausea (with the older compounds) and a lack of controlled studies. An advantage is that pramipexole, ropinirole, and amantadine have been used to treat SSRI-induced sexual dysfunction [45,48]. Both pramipexole and amantadine also may have neuroprotective properties [49], consistent with the neuroprotective/neurogenesis hypothesis of antidepressant action [50,51].

Traditional psychostimulants that affect dopamine as potential augmenting agents include methylphenidate (10–40 mg/d) and dextroamphetamine (5–20 mg/d). Their use has been reported as augmentation of TCAs, MAOIs, and SSRIs [52,53]. The only two controlled trials in TRD were negative [54] (S. Kennedy, personal communication, 2006), and clinicians also may avoid using them because of the potential for abuse by patients who have a history of substance abuse, a frequent comorbid condition with MDD [55]. On the other hand, ADHD is a frequent comorbid condition of MDD [56], and a psychostimulant therefore could be quite helpful [57]. Another disadvantage is that in some cases these agents may worsen cases of anxiety and irritability, and the response may be transient [53]. One clinical advantage is the potential for rapidity of onset of action [58].

A few open trials suggested the efficacy of modafinil (in doses up to 400 mg/d) [59–62]. A double-blind study was positive for the treatment of residual fatigue and sleepiness on SSRIs [63]. A disadvantage of this approach is that its efficacy is unclear in patients who do not experience fatigue and sleepiness. Modafinil is more user friendly than psychostimulants and can be useful for residual symptoms such as fatigue and hypersomnia.

Atypical antipsychotics are being used with increased frequency by clinicians for nonpsychotic MDD. Evidence suggests that risperidone (0.5–2 mg/d) [64,65], olanzapine (5–20 mg/d) [66], ziprasidone (40–80 mg twice daily) [67], quetiapine (25–300 mg/d) [68], and aripiprazole (15–30 mg/d) [69,70] could be efficacious as augmentation agents in TRD. A recent meta-analysis of published and unpublished trials of atypical antipsychotic drug augmentation of antidepressants in TRD suggests that atypical antipsychotics may all have potential antidepressant-augmenting effects [71]. Disadvantages include tolerability (especially, the risk of a metabolic syndrome) and cost. In addition, long-term side effects of the atypical antipsychotics for nonpsychotic MDD are not known. An advantage of this approach is that these drugs may help manage anxiety and agitation.

One of the more innovative sets of augmentations involves compounds related to one carbon metabolism. Folate and related compounds participate in the transfer of methyl groups involved in neurotransmitter synthesis and DNA regulation. Alpert and colleagues [72] found that open augmentation with methylfolate (15–30 mg/d) resulted in a statistically significant improvement in depression scores [72]. The same group found that open addition of s-adenosyl-methionine (SAMe, 800–1600 mg/d) also had promise [73] and currently is conducting two double-blind, placebo-controlled studies in TRD, one of L-methylfolate and one of SAMe. The disadvantages are that there are no controlled studies as yet and that SAMe use is not covered by insurance (because it is an over-the-counter medication). The advantage is that these are naturally occurring substances and often are very acceptable to most patients.

Several anticonvulsants have been studied as augmentation agents. These drugs include lamotrigine (100–300 mg/d) [74,75], gabapentin (300–1800 mg/d) [76], topiramate (100–300 mg/d) [77], carbamazepine (200–400 mg/d) [78], and valproic acid (500–1000 mg/d) [79]. Disadvantages of this approach include potential tolerability issues with some of the anticonvulsants (eg, sedation or weight gain) and the specific risk of Steven Johnson's syndrome with lamotrigine that necessitates a slow dose escalation. A potential advantage is that anticonvulsants may help mitigate anxiety symptoms.

Benzodiazepines may treat anxiety and also help with core depressive symptoms when added to an antidepressant. Evidence exists for the efficacy of lormetazepam in a double-blind, placebo-controlled augmentation study of TCAs [80]. Clonazepam also was nonsignificantly superior to placebo in augmenting fluoxetine [81], and zolpidem was better than placebo in augmenting SSRIs for sleep problems but not depression [82]. The disadvantages include potential sedation and, in the case of benzodiazepines, the possibility of abuse. An advantage is that benzodiazepines may help manage anxiety.

A variety of other augmentation agents have been added to failed trials of antidepressants, but none have been studied extensively. Inositol (up to 12 g/d) was found to be no better than placebo in a double-blind study [83]. Evidence for the opiates oxymorphone [84] and buprenorphine [85] is mostly anecdotal. A small, positive double-blind study supported the use of dehydroepiandrosterone (up to 90 mg/d) [86]. Gonadal hormones have limited support. One small, double-blind study reported positive results from the use of testosterone gel (1% gel, 10 g/d) in men [87], and estrogen has limited support from mostly anecdotal evidence [88].

Combinations

One of the more popular combinations used in clinical practice is an SSRI plus bupropion. Despite its popularity, the evidence for the efficacy of this combination is minimal. Open trials of bupropion (150 mg SR/XL daily or twice daily) initially suggested that this combination would be helpful [89–91]. In a small trial, 54% of 28 partial and nonresponders to SSRIs or venlafaxine responded to an open-label trial of bupropion SR augmentation [92]. A disadvantage of combining SSRIs or serotonin-norepinephrine reuptake inhibitors (SNRIs) with bupropion is tremor [89]. Advantages are the theoretical gain of effecting changes in the dopamine, serotonin, and norepinephrine systems and that the addition of bupropion may help manage SSRI-induced sexual dysfunction [91]. Among citalopram nonresponders in level 2 of the STAR*D study, bupropion combined with citalopram was nonsignificantly more effective than buspirone augmentation [33].

Another intriguing combination of theoretical interest is the dovetailing combination of mirtazapine with SSRIs or with SNRIs. In a placebo-controlled trial of mirtazapine (15–30 mg at night) plus SSRIs, more patients improved with the combination than with placebo addition [93,94]. The considerable promise of the combination resulted in mirtazapine plus the SNRI venlafaxine as being used one of the two treatment options in level 4 of the STAR*D study, in which this combination showed a nonsignificant advantage over tranylcypromine [95]. Disadvantages are the weight gain and sedation associated with the antihistaminergic effects of mirtazapine [93]. Advantages are that mirtazapine plus SSRI should be synergistic: because of its alpha-2 antagonist properties and 5-HT2 and 5-HT3 receptor blocking, mirtazapine could decrease the adverse effects (nausea, anxiety, and sexual dysfunction) caused by SSRI stimulation of these receptors.

In small case series the addition of trazodone or nefazodone to SSRIs was found to result in a positive response rate in patients who had TRD [96–98]. Disadvantages include somnolence (trazodone) and risk of hepatotoxicity (nefazodone). An advantage is that trazodone and nefazodone may help insomnia [99,100].

The combination of SSRIs and TCAs was first reported in 1991 with fluoxetine and desipramine (25–75 mg/d) [101]. Disadvantages are that several SSRIs inhibit the CYP450-2D6 system, and TCAs are substrates of this liver isoenzyme, resulting in increased blood levels of the TCA that can cause more adverse effects or toxicity. Another problem is that low response rates were found in two double-blind studies [20,102]. There is evidence, however, that this combination may produce a more rapid onset of action [103]. Also, remission rates were significantly higher with desipramine plus fluoxetine than with either drug alone [104].

Similar to the combination of SSRIs and TCAs, reboxetine (8–12 mg/d), a norepinephrine uptake inhibitor, has shown some promise [105,106] in combination with SSRIs. Atomoxetine (40–120 mg/d), a norepinephrine reuptake inhibitor (NRI) approved for the treatment of ADHD, was found to be no better than placebo in a large, double-blind trial of TRD [107]. Combining a 5-HT uptake inhibitor and a norepinephrine uptake inhibitor may be useful in severely depressed patients [108]. Also, these NRIs have better safety and tolerability than TCAs.

Switching Pharmacotherapy

If a treatment fails, either because of lack of efficacy or intolerable adverse effects, it makes clinical sense to switch to an alternative treatment. Several choices exist: switching to an alternative pharmacotherapy, switching to an evidence-based psychotherapy, or switching to a neurotherapeutic device that delivers energy to the brain. Pharmacotherapeutic options are reviewed in the next section.

Pharmacotherapy switches for treatment-resistant depression
Many studies of pharmacologic switches have been published, but few are controlled and, at the time of this writing, none includes a placebo comparison. Even with these limitations, the data in aggregate provide an estimate of effectiveness of switching antidepressant medications. Switches can be classified as within or outside of class. Within-class switching has the pharmacologic rationale that each medication shares a common mechanism of action, but each has its own pharmacologic "fingerprint" with differential effects on other neurotransmitters and receptors. Outside-of-class switching is done with the hope that changing the primary mechanism of action will prove more effective.

Switching from one SSRI to another is supported by open trials of "historical failures," showing 50% to 60% response rates when switching from other SSRIs to citalopram [109], from sertraline to fluoxetine [110], or from one SSRI to another [111]. Switching from one SSRI to another may be less effective than switching to a non-SSRI, as suggested by a double-blind study of a switch to paroxetine versus a switch to venlafaxine [112]. The results of level 2 of the STAR*D study showed no significant advantage of switching to a non-SSRI compared with a same-class switch in subjects who had not responded to treatment with one SSRI (citalopram) [113]. An advantage is that the immediate switch from one SSRI to another seems to be well tolerated.

Switching from a TCA to a SSRI is an option that has not received extensive coverage in the literature. A crossover study suggested its efficacy in TCA nonresponders [114]. A prospective trial of sertraline in 12 patients who had TRD and who had not responded to a number of antidepressant trials (n = 7) or who had responded but subsequently suffered a relapse (n = 5) found 41.7% were responders, 8.3% were partial responders, and 50% were nonresponders [115]. The disadvantage of a switch to a SSRI is the well-known high rate of sexual dysfunction in persons treated with SSRIs [116]. An advantage of a SSRI over a TCA is that SSRIs typically are better tolerated than TCAs.

Switching to SNRIs is certainly a reasonable option in TRD. An open study showed 30% to 33% of 84 consecutive patients who had TRD (defined as having not responded to three or more trials) responded to 12 weeks of open treatment with the SNRI venlafaxine (300–450 mg/d) [117]. Similarly, 58% of 152 depressed patients who had not responded to one previous antidepressant trial responded to an 8-week open venlafaxine treatment (75–375 mg/d) [118]. In a larger study, 52.6% of 312 depressed patients who had either "absolute" or "relative" treatment resistance responded to open venlafaxine treatment [119]. Finally, about 69% of 69 SSRI-resistant depressed patients were considered as responders after venlafaxine treatment [120]. Even though a double-blind study found that switching to venlafaxine was significantly superior to a switch to paroxetine (in the observed case analysis) in patients who had TRD [112], the results of level 2 of the STAR*D study did not show any significant advantage of switching citalopram nonresponders to venlafaxine as compared with sertraline [113]. Disadvantages of venlafaxine are blood pressure elevations at higher doses and discontinuation reactions with sudden discontinuation. An advantage is that venlafaxine may be more effective than SSRIs in severe or melancholic depression. An open trial of duloxetine in SSRI-resistant depressed patients showed that the effect size was the same as in patients who were not treatment resistant and started duloxetine [121]. The disadvantage of switching to duloxetine is the lack of controlled studies in TRD.

Switching to mirtazapine is yet another option. Forty-seven percent of patients who had not responded to or tolerated SSRIs showed response to mirtazapine (15–45 mg/d) [122], and 38% responded in another study when patients either were switched to mirtazapine or added it to ongoing medication [94]. The disadvantages of mirtazapine are the adverse effects of sedation and weight gain. The advantages of mirtazapine are that, by blocking 5-HT2 and 5-HT3 receptors, mirtazapine may prevent SSRI discontinuation–emergent adverse events, and immediate switching seems to be well tolerated [122].

Switching to bupropion is an opportunity to expose patients to the novel dual mechanism of norepinephrine and dopamine uptake inhibition. The first report of bupropion switch was in 1983. Among 30 TCA nonresponders, bupropion was better than placebo in reducing depressive symptoms [123]. Sixty-one patients who had not responded to at least one antidepressant and who then took either citalopram or bupropion for 6 weeks and did not respond were switched to the alternative medication or to citalopram combined with bupropion. Switching resulted in a remission rate of 7%; 28% reached remission with the combination [124]. A disadvantage of switching from an SSRI to bupropion is that SSRI-induced discontinuation reactions may occur [125]. An advantage is that a switch to bupropion reduces the incidence of weight gain and sexual dysfunction associated with SSRIs [126,127]. The results of level 2 of the STAR*D study did not show any difference in remission rates among citalopram nonresponders switched to bupropion and those switched to venlafaxine and sertraline [113].

Clinical lore suggests that the older generation of TCAs may have greater efficacy than SSRIs, but the literature on such a switch is small. A few studies found some efficacy with a switch to a TCA in patients who had TRD and in SSRI nonresponders [114,128,129]. The disadvantages are the usual side effects and toxicity caused by TCAs: sedation, anticholinergic side effects, weight gain, and lethality in overdose. Advantages include a clear dose–response curve, the low cost of some of the generic TCAs, and possible superiority of some TCAs compared with SSRIs in severe/melancholic depression [130–132].

Nefazodone and trazodone are two antidepressants that are used frequently for insomnia; data clearly support their antidepressant efficacy. In terms of switching, a retrospective study of 20 depressed patients who had not responded to or tolerated prior antidepressant treatment suggested the usefulness of trazodone [133]. Patients who had discontinued an SSRI because of "poor response" showed significant improvement with nefazodone (300–600 mg/d) [134]. The disadvantages are that these medications frequently are underdosed, and nefazodone requires twice-daily dosing. Furthermore, nefazodone has a black box warning because of the risk of fatal hepatic toxicity. Advantages include less weight gain and sexual dysfunction than seen with SSRIs [127,135].

MAOIs are used less frequently but also can be considered as alternative agents for switching. In one study of patients who had not responded to imipramine, 58% to 65% showed improvement with MAOIs [136,137]. Disadvantages include dietary restrictions, risk of hypertensive crises and serotonin syndromes, and the need for wash-outs before starting and after ending treatment. Advantages are that the MAOIs are useful in atypical unipolar depression [138] and anergic bipolar depression. The considerable promise of the MAOIs in TRD resulted in the choice of tranylcypromine as one of the two treatment options in level 4 of the STAR*D study, in which it was found to be nonsignificantly less effective than the mirtazapine/venlafaxine combination [95].

The norepinephrine uptake inhibitors reboxetine (4–10 mg/d) [139] and atomoxetine (40–120 mg/d) [140] also may have some usefulness as switching agents. In one study, patients who had not responded to an adequate trial with fluoxetine showed significant improvement with open reboxetine (8–10 mg/d) [139]. Disadvantages are that switching from an SSRI with a short half-life requires tapering and that no studies with atomoxetine have been reported in TRD. Reboxetine is not approved by the Food and Drug Administration (although it is approved in Europe). Advantages are that the norepinephrine uptake inhibitors are potentially useful in SSRI nonresponders who have a history of prior TCA response and perhaps in patients who have MDD with comorbid ADHD.

LONG-TERM FINDINGS OF THE SEQUENCED TREATMENT ALTERNATIVES TO RELIEVE DEPRESSION STUDY

The STAR*D study [17,18] was designed to assess the relative effectiveness of competing treatments for patients who had MDD and who did not reach remission with an initial trial of citalopram. The results of the study have been summarized elsewhere [15]. Because of the design using equipoise randomization, after failure to remit with a vigorous trial of measurement-based treatment with citalopram, patients were assigned randomly to either switching or augmentation strategies.

As mentioned earlier, initial switching strategies showed that about 30% of patients reached remission with a switch to another SSRI (sertraline), to an SNRI (venlafaxine), or to a norepinephrine/dopamine uptake blocker (bupropion). This result shows that mechanism of action is less important than predicted and allows clinicians to choose the medication that best fits the patient in terms of adverse-effect profile. If patients did not reach remission after this switch, they could be assigned randomly to either switching or augmentation for yet another level of treatment. Those who were assigned randomly to switching could take either the TCA nortriptyline or the unique medication mirtazapine. Here the results were more modest, with about 15% reaching remission and without any statistically significant difference between switching options [141]. Patients who still did not reach remission and who were willing to continue in the study then were switched to either the combination of venlafaxine and mirtazapine or to the MAOI tranylcypromine. Again, the results were modest, with about 13% reaching remission; patients discontinued tranylcypromine more frequently than the combination of venlafaxine and mirtazapine.

As for STAR*D augmentation or combination options, patients who did not reach remission with citalopram treatment could be assigned randomly to augment ongoing citalopram with bupropion or buspirone. Both augmentations resulted in about one third of patients reaching remission, but bupropion was better tolerated [113]. Patients who did not reach remission after the second level of treatment were assigned randomly to either lithium or thyroid. About 15% of patients reached remission overall, but patients tolerated thyroid better than lithium, and the remission rates on thyroid were nonsignificantly higher (24%) [22].

In one of the few follow-up studies of TRD, patients who reached remission after any level in the STAR*D study were followed for up to a year [15]. About 50% of those who exited level 1 treatment with citalopram relapsed within 12 months. Seventy percent of those who exited level 2 and about 80% for those who exited level 3 relapsed. Furthermore, those who reached remission fared better than those who responded but did not reach remission. These data indicate that the long-term management of TRD remains a challenge.

References

[1] Kessler RC, Berglund P, Demler O, et al. Lifetime prevalence and age-of-onset distributions of DSM-IV disorders in the National Comorbidity Survey Replication. Arch Gen Psychiatry 2005;62(6):593–602.

[2] Kessler RC, Chiu WT, Demler O, et al. Prevalence, severity, and comorbidity of 12-month DSM-IV disorders in the National Comorbidity Survey Replication. Arch Gen Psychiatry 2005;62:617–27.

[3] Wang PS, Berglund P, Olfson M, et al. Failure and delay in initial treatment contact after first onset of mental disorders in the National Comorbidity Survey Replication. Arch Gen Psychiatry 2005;62(6):603–13.

[4] Kessler RC, Akiskal HS, Ames M, et al. Prevalence and effects of mood disorders on work performance in a nationally representative sample of U.S. workers. Am J Psychiatry 2006;163(9):1561–8.

[5] Wang PS, Lane M, Olfson M, et al. Twelve-month use of mental health services in the United States: results from the National Comorbidity Survey Replication. Arch Gen Psychiatry 2005;62(6):629–40.

[6] Rush AJ, Kraemer HC, Sackeim HA, et al. Report by the ACNP Task Force on response and remission in major depressive disorder. Neuropsychopharmacology 2006;31(9):1841–53.

[7] Fava M, Davidson KG. Definition and epidemiology of treatment-resistant depression. Psychiatr Clin North Am 1996;19(2):179–200.

[8] Simon GE, Khandker RK, Ichikawa L, et al. Recovery from depression predicts lower health services costs. J Clin Psychiatry 2006;67(8):1226–31.
[9] Judd LL, Akiskal HS, Maser JD, et al. Major depressive disorder: a prospective study of residual subthreshold depressive symptoms as predictor of rapid relapse. J Affect Disord 1998;50:97–108.
[10] Judd LL, Akiskal HS, Maser JD, et al. A prospective 12-year study of subsyndromal and syndromal depressive symptoms in unipolar major depressive disorders. Arch Gen Psychiatry 1998;55:694–700.
[11] Kessler RC, Berglund P, Demler O, et al. The epidemiology of major depressive disorder. JAMA 2003;289(23):3095–105.
[12] Sheehan DV, Lecrubier Y, Sheehan KH, et al. The Mini-International Neuropsychiatric Interview (M.I.N.I.): the development and validation of a structured diagnostic psychiatric interview for DSM-IV and ICD-10. J Clin Psychiatry 1998;59(Suppl 20):22–33.
[13] Spitzer R, Williams J, First MGM. Structured clinical interview for DSM-IV-patient edition (SCID-P, 9/1/1989 version). New York: Biometrics Research Department, New York State Psychiatric Institute; 1989.
[14] Zimmerman M, Mattia JI. The reliability and validity of a screening questionnaire for 13 DSM-IV axis I disorders (the Psychiatric Diagnostic Screening Questionnaire) in psychiatric outpatients. J Clin Psychiatry 1999;60(10):677–83.
[15] Rush AJ, Trivedi MH, Wisniewski SR, et al. Acute and longer-term outcomes in depressed outpatients requiring one or several treatment steps: a STAR*D report. Am J Psychiatry 2006;163(11):1905–17.
[16] Fava M. Diagnosis and definition of treatment-resistant depression. Biol Psychiatry 2003;53(8):649–59.
[17] Rush AJ, Fava M, Wisniewski SR, et al. Sequenced treatment alternatives to relieve depression (STAR*D): rationale and design. Control Clin Trials 2004;25(1):119–42.
[18] Fava M, Rush AJ, Trivedi MH, et al. Background and rationale for the sequenced treatment alternatives to relieve depression (STAR*D) study. Psychiatr Clin North Am 2003;26(2):457–94.
[19] Bauer M, Dopfmer S. Lithium augmentation treatment-resistant depression: meta-analysis of placebo-controlled studies. J Clin Psychopharmacol 1999;19(5):427–34.
[20] Fava M, Alpert J, Nierenberg A, et al. Double-blind study of high-dose fluoxetine versus lithium or desipramine augmentation of fluoxetine in partial responders and nonresponders to fluoxetine. J Clin Psychopharmacol 2002;22(4):379–87.
[21] Nierenberg AA, Papakostas GI, Petersen T, et al. Lithium augmentation of nortriptyline for subjects resistant to multiple antidepressants. J Clin Psychopharmacol 2003;23(1):92–5.
[22] Nierenberg AA, Fava M, Trivedi MH, et al. A comparison of lithium and T(3) augmentation following two failed medication treatments for depression: a STAR*D report. Am J Psychiatry 2006;163(9):1519–30.
[23] Salama AA, Shafey M. A case of severe lithium toxicity induced by combined fluoxetine and lithium carbonate. Am J Psychiatry 1989;146(2):278.
[24] Valenstein M, McCarthy JF, Austin KL, et al. What happened to lithium? Antidepressant augmentation in clinical settings. Am J Psychiatry 2006;163(7):1219–25.
[25] Aronson R, Offman HJ, Joffe RT, et al. Triiodothyronine augmentation in the treatment of refractory depression: a meta-analysis. Arch Gen Psychiatry 1996;53(9):842–8.
[26] Joffe RT, Singer W. A comparison of triiodothyronine and thyroxine in the potentiation of tricyclic antidepressants. Psychiatry Res 1990;32(3):241–51.
[27] Agid O, Lerer B. Algorithm-based treatment of major depression in an outpatient clinic: clinical correlates of response to a specific serotonin reuptake inhibitor and to triiodothyronine augmentation. Int J Neuropsychopharmacol 2003;6(1):41–9.
[28] Clayton AH, Shen C. T4 augmentation in partial responders with major depression. Presented at the annual meeting of the New Clinical Drug Evaluation Unit (NCDEU). Boca Raton (FL), June 10–13, 2002.

[29] Iosifescu DV, Nierenberg AA, Mischoulon D, et al. An open study of triiodothyronine augmentation of selective serotonin reuptake inhibitors in treatment-resistant major depressive disorder. J Clin Psychiatry 2005;66(8):1038–42.

[30] Dimitriou EC, Dimitriou CE. Buspirone augmentation of antidepressant therapy. J Clin Psychopharmacol 1998;18(6):465–9.

[31] Landen M, Bjorling G, Agren H, et al. A randomized, double-blind, placebo-controlled trial of buspirone in combination with an SSRI in patients with treatment-refractory depression. J Clin Psychiatry 1998;59(12):664–8.

[32] Appelberg BG, Syvalahti EK, Koskinen TE, et al. Patients with severe depression may benefit from buspirone augmentation of selective serotonin reuptake inhibitors: results from placebo-controlled, randomized, double-blind, placebo wash-in study. J Clin Psychiatry 2001;62(6):448–52.

[33] Trivedi MH, Fava M, Wisniewski SR, et al. Medication augmentation after the failure of SSRIs for depression. N Engl J Med 2006;354(12):1243–52.

[34] Landen M, Erikkson E, Agren H, et al. Effect of buspirone on sexual dysfunction in depressed patients treated with selective serotonin reuptake inhibitors. J Clin Psychopharmacol 1999;19(3):268–71.

[35] Blier P, Bergeron B. The use of pindolol to potentiate antidepressant medication. J Clin Psychiatry 1998;59(Suppl 5):16–23.

[36] Rabiner EA, Bhagwagar Z, Gunn RN, et al. Pindolol augmentation of selective serotonin reuptake inhibitors: PET evidence that the dose used in clinical trials is too low. Am J Psychiatry 2001;158(12):2080–2.

[37] Moreno FA, Gelenberh AJ, Bachar K, et al. Pindolol augmentation of treatment-resistant depressed patients. J Clin Psychiatry 1997;58(10):437–9.

[38] Perez V, Soler J, Puigdemont D, et al. A double-blind, randomized, placebo-controlled, trial of pindolol augmentation in depressive patients resistant to serotonin reuptake inhibitors. Grup de Recerca en Trastorns Afectius. Arch Gen Psychiatry 1999;56(4):375–9.

[39] Perry EB, Berman RM, Sanacora G, et al. Pindolol augmentation in depressed patients resistant to selective serotonin reuptake inhibitors: a double-blind, randomized, controlled trial. J Clin Psychiatry 2004;65(2):238–43.

[40] Blier P, Bergeron B. Effectiveness of pindolol with selected antidepressant drugs in the treatment of major depression. J Clin Psychopharmacol 1995;15(3):217–22.

[41] Ballesteros J, Callado LF. Effectiveness of pindolol plus serotonin uptake inhibitors in depression: a meta-analysis of early and late outcomes from randomized controlled trials. J Affect Disord 2004;79(1–3):137–47.

[42] Bouckoms A, Mangini L. Pergolide: an antidepressant adjuvant for mood disorders? Psychopharmacol Bull 1993;29(2):207–11.

[43] Izumi T, Inoue T, Kitagawa N, et al. Open pergolide treatment of tricyclic and heterocyclic antidepressant-resistant depression. J Affect Disord 2000;61(1–2):127–32.

[44] Stryjer R, Strous RD, Shaked G, et al. Amantadine as augmentation therapy in the management of treatment-resistant depression. Int Clin Psychopharmacol 2003;18(2):93–6.

[45] Sporn J, Ghaemi SN, Sambur MR, et al. Pramipexole augmentation in the treatment of unipolar and bipolar depression: a retrospective chart review. Ann Clin Psychiatry 2000; 12(3):137–40.

[46] Lattanzi L, Dell'Osso L, Cassano P, et al. Pramipexole in treatment-resistant depression: a 16-week naturalistic study. Bipolar Disord 2002;4(5):307–14.

[47] Perugi G, Toni C, Ruffalo G, et al. Adjunctive dopamine agonists in treatment-resistant bipolar II depression: an open case series. Pharmacopsychiatry 2001;34(4):137–41.

[48] Michelson D, Bancroft J, Targum S, et al. Female sexual dysfunction associated with antidepressant administration: a randomized, placebo-controlled study of pharmacologic intervention. Am J Psychiatry 2000;157(2):239–43.

[49] Du F, Li R, Huang Y, et al. Dopamine D3 receptor-preferring agonists induce neurotrophic effects on mesencephalic dopamine neurons. Eur J Neurosci 2005;22(10):2422–30.

[50] Duman RS. Role of neurotrophic factors in the etiology and treatment of mood disorders. Neuromolecular Med 2004;5(1):11–25.
[51] Santarelli L, Saxe M, Gross C, et al. Requirement of hippocampal neurogenesis for the behavioral effects of antidepressants. Science 2003;301(5634):805–9.
[52] Warneke L. Psychostimulants in psychiatry. Can J Psychiatry 1990;35(1):3–10.
[53] Fawcett J, Kravitz HM, Zajecka JM, et al. CNS stimulant potentiation of monoamine oxidase inhibitors in treatment-refractory depression. J Clin Psychopharmacol 1991;11(2): 127–32.
[54] Patkar AA, Masand PS, Pae CU, et al. A randomized, double-blind, placebo-controlled trial of augmentation with an extended release formulation of methylphenidate in outpatients with treatment-resistant depression. J Clin Psychopharmacol 2006;26(6):653–6.
[55] Davis LL, Frazier E, Husain MM, et al. Substance use disorder comorbidity in major depressive disorder: a confirmatory analysis of the STAR*D cohort. Am J Addict 2006;15(4): 278–85.
[56] Alpert JE, Maddocks A, Nierenberg AA, et al. Attention deficit hyperactivity disorder in childhood among adults with major depression. Psychiatry Res 1996;62(3):213–9.
[57] Findling RL. Open-label treatment of comorbid depression and attentional disorders with co-administration of serotonin reuptake inhibitors and psychostimulants in children, adolescents, and adults: a case series. J Child Adolesc Psychopharmacol 1996;6(3): 165–75.
[58] Lavretsky H, Kim MD, Kumar A, et al. Combined treatment with methylphenidate and citalopram for accelerated response in the elderly: an open trial. J Clin Psychiatry 2003; 64(12):1410–4.
[59] Menza MA, Kaufman KR, Castellanos A. Modafinil augmentation of antidepressant treatment in depression. J Clin Psychiatry 2000;61(5):378–81.
[60] DeBattista C, Lembke A, Solvason HB, et al. A prospective trial of modafinil as an adjunctive treatment of major depression. J Clin Psychopharmacol 2004;24(1):87–90.
[61] Kogeorgos J, Kotrotsou M, Polonifis N, et al. Modafinil as augmentation of antidepressant therapy. Eur Neuropsychopharmacol 2002;12(s3):S211–2.
[62] Schwartz TL, Leso L, Beale M, et al. Modafinil in the treatment of depression with severe comorbid medical illness. Psychosomatics 2002;43(3):336–7.
[63] Fava M, Thase ME, DeBattista C. A multicenter, placebo-controlled study of modafinil augmentation in partialresponders to selective serotonin reuptake inhibitors with persistent fatigue and sleepiness. J Clin Psychiatry 2005;66(1):85–93.
[64] Ostroff RB, Nelson JC. Risperidone augmentation of selective serotonin reuptake inhibitors in major depression. J Clin Psychiatry 1999;60(4):256–9.
[65] Rapaport MH, Gharabawi GM, Canuso CM, et al. Effects of risperidone augmentation in patients with treatment-resistant depression: Results of open-label treatment followed by double-blind continuation. Neuropsychopharmacology 2006;31(11):2505–13.
[66] Shelton RC, Tollefson GD, Tohen M, et al. A novel augmentation strategy for treating resistant major depression. Am J Psychiatry 2001;158(1):131–4.
[67] Papakostas G, Petersen TJ, Nierenberg AA, et al. Ziprasidone augmentation of selective serotonin reuptake inhibitors (SSRIs) for SSRI-resistant major depressive disorder. J Clin Psychiatry 2004;65(2):217–21.
[68] Adson DE, Kushner MG, Eiben KM, et al. Preliminary experience with adjunctive quetiapine in patients receiving selective serotonin reuptake inhibitors. Depress Anxiety 2004; 19(2):121–6.
[69] Worthington JJ 3rd, Kinrys G, Wygant LE, et al. Aripiprazole as an augmentor of selective serotonin reuptake inhibitors in depression and anxiety disorder patients. Int Clin Psychopharmacol 2005;20(1):9–11.
[70] Papakostas GI, Petersen TJ, Kinrys G, et al. Aripiprazole augmentation of selective serotonin reuptake inhibitors for treatment-resistant major depressive disorder. J Clin Psychiatry 2005;66(10):1326–30.

[71] Papakostas G, Shelton R, Fava M. Augmentation with atypical antipsychotic agents for treatment-resistant major depressive disorder: a meta-analysis of double-blind, placebo-controlled studies. J Clin Psychiatry, in press.

[72] Alpert JE, Mischoulon D, Rubenstein GE, et al. Folinic acid (leucovorin) as an adjunctive treatment for SSRI-refractory depression. Ann Clin Psychiatry 2002;14(1):33–8.

[73] Alpert JE, Papakostas G, Mischoulon D, et al. S-adenosyl-L-methionine (SAMe) as an adjunct for resistant major depressive disorder: an open trial following partial or nonresponse to selective reuptake inhibitors or venlafaxine. J Clin Psychopharmacol 2004; 24(6):661.

[74] Rocha FL, Hara C. Lamotrigine augmentation in unipolar depression. Int Clin Psychopharmacol 2003;18(2):97–9.

[75] Barbee JG, Jamhour NJ. Lamotrigine as an augmentation agent in treatment-resistant depression. J Clin Psychiatry 2002;63(8):737–41.

[76] Yasmin S, Carpenter LL, Leon Z, et al. Adjunctive gabapentin in treatment-resistant depression: a retrospective chart review. J Affect Disord 2001;63(1–3):243–7.

[77] Schmidt do Prado-Lima PA, Bacaltchuck J. Topiramate in treatment-resistant depression and binge-eating disorder. Bipolar Disord 2002;4(4):271–3.

[78] Otani K, Yasui N, Kaneko S, et al. Carbamazepine augmentation therapy in three patients with trazodone-resistant unipolar depression. Int Clin Psychopharmacol 1996;11(1): 55–7.

[79] Hantouche EG, Akiskal HS, Lancrenon S, et al. Mood stabilizer augmentation in apparently « unipolar » MDD: predictors of response in the naturalistic French national EPIDEP study. J Affect Disord 2005;84(2–3):243–9.

[80] Nolen WA, Haffmans PM, Bouvy PF, et al. Hypnotics as concurrent medication in depression: a placebo-controlled, double-blind comparison of flunitrazepam and lormetazepam in patients with major depression, treated with a (tri) cyclic antidepressant. J Affect Disord 1993;28(3):179–88.

[81] Smith WT, Londborg PD, Glaudin V, et al. Short-term augmentation of fluoxetine with clonazepam in the treatment of depression: a double-blind study. Am J Psychiatry 1998;155(10):1339–45.

[82] Asnis GM, Chakraburtty A, DuBoff EA, et al. Zolpidem for persistent insomnia in SSRI-treated depressed patients. J Clin Psychiatry 1999;60(10):668–76.

[83] Nemets B, Mishory A, Levine J, et al. Inositol addition does not improve depression in SSRI treatment failure. J Neural Transm 1999;106(7–8):795–8.

[84] Stoll AL, Rueter S. Treatment augmentation with opiates in severe and refractory major depression. Am J Psychiatry 1999;156(12):2017.

[85] Bodkin JA, Zornberg GL, Lukas SE, et al. Buprenorphine treatment of refractory depression. J Clin Psychopharmacol 1995;15(1):49–57.

[86] Wolkowitz OM, Reus VI, Keebler A, et al. Double-blind treatment of major depression with dehydroepiandrosterone. Am J Psychiatry 1999;156(4):646–9.

[87] Pope HG Jr, Cohane GH, Kanayama G, et al. Testosterone gel supplementation for men with refractory depression: a randomized, placebo-controlled trial. Am J Psychiatry 2003; 160(1):105–11.

[88] Stahl SM. Natural estrogen as an antidepressant for women. J Clin Psychiatry 2001;62(6): 404–5.

[89] Bodkin JA, Lasser RA, Wines JD Jr, et al. Combining serotonin reuptake inhibitors and bupropion in partial responders to antidepressant monotherapy. J Clin Psychiatry 1997;58(4):137–45.

[90] Ramasubbu R. Treatment of resistant depression by adding noradrenergic agents to lithium augmentation of SSRIs. Ann Pharmacother 2002;36(4):634–40.

[91] Kennedy SH, McCann SM, Masellis M, et al. Combining bupropion SR with venlafaxine, paroxetine, or fluoxetine: a preliminary report on pharmacokinetic, therapeutic, and sexual dysfunction effects. J Clin Psychiatry 2002;63(3):181–6.

[92] DeBattista C, Solvason HB, Poirier J, et al. A prospective trial of bupropion SR augmentation of partial and non-responders to serotonergic antidepressants. J Clin Psychopharmacol 2003;23(1):27–30.

[93] Carpenter LL, Yasmin S, Price LH. A double-blind, placebo-controlled study of antidepressant augmentation with mirtazapine. Biol Psychiatry 2002;51(2):183–8.

[94] Wan DD, Kundhur D, Solomons K, et al. Mirtazapine for treatment-resistant depression: a preliminary report. J Psychiatry Neurosci 2003;28(1):55–9.

[95] McGrath PJ, Stewart JW, Fava M, et al. Tranylcypromine versus venlafaxine plus mirtazapine following three failed antidepressant medication trials for depression: a STAR*D report. Am J Psychiatry 2006;163(9):1531–41.

[96] Dam J, Ryde L, Svejso J, et al. Morning fluoxetine plus evening mianserin versus morning fluoxetine plus evening placebo in the acute treatment of major depression. Pharmacopsychiatry 1998;31(2):48–54.

[97] Maes M, Libbrecht I, van Hundel F, et al. Pindolol and mianserin augment the antidepressant activity of fluoxetine in hospitalized major depressed patients, including those with treatment resistance. J Clin Psychopharmacol 1999;19(2):177–82.

[98] Ferreri M, Lavergne F, Berlin I, et al. Benefits from mianserin augmentation of fluoxetine in patients with major depression non-responders to fluoxetine alone. Acta Psychiatr Scand 2001;103(1):66–72.

[99] Nierenberg AA, Keck PE Jr. Management of monoamine oxidase inhibitor-associated insomnia with trazodone. J Clin Psychopharmacol 1989;9(1):42–5.

[100] Nierenberg AA, Adler LA, Peselow E, et al. Trazodone for antidepressant-associated insomnia. Am J Psychiatry 1994;151(7):1069–72.

[101] Weilburg JB, Rosenbaum JF, Meltzer-Brody S, et al. Tricyclic augmentation of fluoxetine. Ann Clin Psychiatry 1991;3:209–13.

[102] Fava M, Rosenbaum JF, McGrath PJ, et al. Lithium and tricyclic augmentation of fluoxetine treatment for resistant major depression: a double-blind, controlled study. Am J Psychiatry 1994;15(9):1372–4.

[103] Nelson JC, Mazure CM, Bowers MB Jr, et al. A preliminary, open study of the combination of fluoxetine and desipramine for rapid treatment of major depression. Arch Gen Psychiatry 1991;48:303–7.

[104] Nelson JC, Mazure CM, Jatlow PI, et al. Combining norepinephrine and serotonin reuptake inhibition mechanisms for treatment of depression: a double-blind, randomized study. Biol Psychiatry 2004;55(3):296–300.

[105] Hawley CJ, Sivakumaran T, Ochocki M, et al. Co-administration of reboxetine and serotonin selective reuptake inhibitors in treatment-resistant patients with major depression. Presented at the 39th annual meeting of the American College of Neuropsychopharmacology (ACNP). San Juan (PR), December 10–14, 2000.

[106] Dursun SM, Devarajan S. Reboxetine plus citalopram for refractory depression not responding to venlafaxine: possible mechanisms. Psychopharmacology (Berl) 2001; 153(4):497–8.

[107] Michaelson, et al. CINP 2006.

[108] Nelson JC. Augmentation strategies with serotonergic-noradrenergic combinations. J Clin Psychiatry 1998;59(Suppl 5):65–8.

[109] Thase ME, Feighner JP, Lydiard RB. Citalopram treatment of fluoxetine nonresponders. J Clin Psychiatry 2001;62:683–7.

[110] Thase ME, Blomgren SL, Birkett MA, et al. Fluoxetine treatment of patients with major depressive disorder who failed initial treatment with sertraline. J Clin Psychiatry 1997;58: 16–21.

[111] Joffe RT, Levitt AJ, Sokolov ST, et al. Response to an open trial of a second SSRI in major depression. J Clin Psychiatry 1996;57:114–5.

[112] Poirier MF, Boyer P. Venlafaxine and paroxetine in treatment-resistant depression: double-blind, randomized comparison. Br J Psychiatry 1999;175:12–6.

[113] Rush AJ, Trivedi MH, Wisniewski SR, et al. Bupropion-SR, sertraline, or venlafaxine-XR after failure of SSRIs for depression. N Engl J Med 2006;354(12):1231–42.

[114] Thase ME, Rush AJ, Howland RH, et al. Double-blind switch study of imipramine or sertraline treatment of antidepressant-resistant chronic depression. Arch Gen Psychiatry 2002; 59(3):233–9.

[115] Papakostas GI, Petersen T, Worthington JJ, et al. A pilot, open study of sertraline in outpatients with treatment-resistant depression (TRD) or with a history of TRD who responded but later relapsed. Int Clin Psychopharmacol 2003;18(5):293–6.

[116] Clayton AH, Pradko JF, Croft HA, et al. Prevalence of sexual dysfunction among newer antidepressants. J Clin Psychiatry 2002;63(4):357–66.

[117] Nierenberg AA, Feighner JP, Rudolph R, et al. Venlafaxine for treatment-resistant unipolar depression. J Clin Psychopharmacol 1994;14:419–23.

[118] de Montigny C, Silverstone PH, Debonnel G, et al. Venlafaxine in treatment-resistant major depression: a Canadian multicenter, open-label trial. J Clin Psychopharmacol 1999;19: 401–6.

[119] Mitchell PB, Schweitzer I, Burrows G, et al. Efficacy of venlafaxine and predictors of response in a prospective open-label study of patients with treatment-resistant major depression. J Clin Psychopharmacol 2000;20(4):483–7.

[120] Saiz-Ruiz J, Ibanez A, Diaz-Marsa M, et al. Efficacy of venlafaxine in major depression resistant to selective serotonin reuptake inhibitors. Prog Neuropsychopharmacol Biol Psychiatry 2002;26(6):1129–34.

[121] Wohlreich MM, Mallinckrodt CH, Watkin JG, et al. Immediate switching of antidepressant therapy: results from a clinical trial of duloxetine. Ann Clin Psychiatry 2005;17(4): 259–68.

[122] Fava M, Dunner DL, Greist JH, et al. Efficacy and safety of mirtazapine in major depressive disorder patients after SSRI treatment failure: an open-label trial. J Clin Psychiatry 2001; 62(6):413–20.

[123] Stern WC, Harto-Truax N, Bauer N. Efficacy of bupropion in tricyclic-resistant or intolerant patients. J Clin Psychiatry 1983;44(5 Pt 2):148–52.

[124] Lam RW, Hossie H, Solomons K, et al. Citalopram and bupropion-SR: combining versus switching in patients with treatment-resistant depression. J Clin Psychiatry 2004;65(3): 337–40.

[125] Clayton AH, McGarvey EL, Abouesh AI, et al. Substitution of an SSRI with bupropion sustained release following SSRI-induced sexual dysfunction. J Clin Psychiatry 2001;62(3): 185–90.

[126] Kavoussi RJ, Segraves RT, Hughes AR, et al. Double-blind comparison of bupropion sustained release and sertraline in depressed outpatients. J Clin Psychiatry 1997;58(12): 532–7.

[127] Fava M. Weight gain and antidepressants. J Clin Psychiatry 2000;61(Suppl 11): 37–41.

[128] Weintraub D. Nortriptyline in geriatric depression resistant to serotonin reuptake inhibitors: case series. J Geriatr Psychiatry Neurol 2001;14(1):28–32.

[129] Nierenberg AA, Papakostas GI, Petersen T, et al. Nortriptyline for treatment-resistant depression. J Clin Psychiatry 2003;64(1):35–9.

[130] Anderson IM. Selective serotonin reuptake inhibitors versus tricyclic antidepressants: a meta-analysis of efficacy and tolerability. J Affect Disord 2000;58(1):19–36.

[131] Danish University Antidepressant Group. Citalopram: clinical effect profile in comparison with clomipramine. A controlled multicenter study. Psychopharmacology (Berl) 1986; 90(1):131–8.

[132] Danish University Antidepressant Group. Paroxetine: a selective serotonin reuptake inhibitor showing better tolerance, but weaker antidepressant effect than clomipramine in a controlled multicenter study. J Affect Disord 1990;18(4):289–99.

[133] Sajatovic M, DiGiovanni S, Fuller M, et al. Nefazodone therapy in patients with treatment-resistant or treatment-intolerant depression and high psychiatric comorbidity. Clin Ther 1999;21:733–40.

[134] Thase ME, Zajecka J, Kornstein SG, et al. Nefazodone treatment of patients with poor response to SSRIS. Presented at the 37th annual meeting of the American College of Neuropsychopharmacology (ACNP). Las Croabas (PR), December 14–18, 1998.

[135] Feiger A, Kiev A, Shrivastava RK, et al. Nefazodone versus sertraline in outpatients with major depression:focus on efficacy, tolerability, and effects on sexual function and satisfaction. J Clin Psychiatry 1996;57(Suppl 2):53–62.

[136] McGrath PJ, Stewart JW, Harrison W, et al. Treatment of tricyclic refractory depression with a monoamine oxidase inhibitor antidepressant. Psychopharmacol Bull 1987;23: 169–72.

[137] Thase ME, Mallinger AG, McKnight D, et al. Treatment of imipramine-resistant recurrent depression, IV: a double-blind crossover study of tranylcypromine for anergic bipolar depression. Am J Psychiatry 1992;149:195–8.

[138] Quitkin FM, Stewart JW, McGrath PJ, et al. Columbia atypical depression: a subgroup of depressives with better response to MAOI than to tricyclic antidepressants or placebo. Br J Psychiatry Suppl 1993;21:30–4.

[139] Fava M, McGrath PJ, Sheu WP. Reboxetine Study Group. Switching to reboxetine: an efficacy and safety study in patients with major depressive disorder unresponsive to fluoxetine. J Clin Psychopharmacol 2003;23(4):365–9.

[140] Chouinard G, Annable L, Bradwejn J. An early phase II clinical trial of tomoxetine (LY139603) in the treatment of newly admitted depressed patients. Psychopharmacology (Berl) 1984;83(1):126–8.

[141] Fava M, Rush AJ, Wisniewski SR, et al. A comparison of mirtazapine and nortriptyline following two consecutive failed medication treatments for depressed outpatients: a STAR*D report. Am J Psychiatry 2006;163(7):1161–72.

Somatic Therapies for Treatment-Resistant Depression: New Neurotherapeutic Interventions

Darin D. Dougherty, MD[a],*, Scott L. Rauch, MD[b]

[a]Department of Psychiatry, Massachusetts General Hospital, 15 Parkman Street, Boston, MA 02114, USA
[b]Department of Psychiatry, McLean Hospital, 115 Mill Street, Belmont, MA 02478, USA

The most commonly used treatments for major depressive episodes are pharmacotherapy and psychotherapy. Although the majority of patients suffering from a major depressive episode improve significantly with these treatments, a minority does not achieve adequate symptom reduction; this minority is described as having treatment-resistant depression (TRD). The largest study of treatment response and relapse ever conducted, the Sequenced Treatment Alternatives to Relieve Depression (STAR*D), found that with each failed medication trial the remission rate decreased, the relapse rate increased, and the time to relapse decreased [1]. Although the definition of TRD is imperfect, the STAR*D data suggest that patients who have major depression and who have failed to respond to three or four medication trials are treatment resistant.

Until recently, few treatments for major depression other than pharmacotherapy, psychotherapy, and electroconvulsive therapy (ECT) have been available. This article reviews recent data from the field of somatic therapies for TRD. These new treatments are device-related and/or surgical interventions for major depression and other psychiatric illnesses, and the field associated with these new treatments often is referred to as "neurotherapeutics" or "neuromodulation." These treatments are typically (but not always) used in TRD patients. Examples of neurotherapeutic interventions for major depression include ablative limbic system surgeries (eg, anterior cingulotomy and subcaudate tractotomy), vagus nerve stimulation (VNS), transcranial magnetic stimulation (TMS), and deep brain stimulation (DBS). Although this review should not be considered a comprehensive overview, it briefly discusses the role of

Dr. Dougherty has received research support from Cyberonics, Medtronic, and Northstar Neuroscience and has received speaking honoraria from Cyberonics.

Dr. Rauch has received research support from Cyberonics, Medtronic, and Cephalon, fellowship support from Pfizer, and honoraria from Cyberonics and Novartis.

*Corresponding author. E-mail address: ddougherty@partners.org (D.D. Dougherty).

0193-953X/07/$ – see front matter
doi:10.1016/j.psc.2006.12.006

each of these neurotherapeutic interventions in treating depression. It concludes with thoughts on the future potential of neurotherapeutic interventions in the treatment of depression.

ELECTROCONVULSIVE THERAPY

ECT has been used to treat depression since the 1930s, and it is used commonly today to treat patients who have TRD. ECT is administered by delivering electrical current to the brain through the scalp and skull, in either a unilateral or bilateral manner, to induce a generalized seizure. Although the mechanism of action is incompletely understood, the efficacy of ECT for depression has been demonstrated in a large number of clinical trials. A recent review and meta-analysis found that real ECT was significantly more effective than simulated ECT (six trials, 256 patients), and treatment with ECT was significantly more effective than pharmacotherapy (18 trials, 1144 patients) [2]. In this same analysis bilateral ECT was more effective than unipolar ECT (22 trials, 1408 participants) [2]. Patients often require continued maintenance treatments, however, and significant side effects such as memory loss are associated with ECT [3].

ABLATIVE LIMBIC SYSTEM SURGERY

Ablative neurosurgery for psychiatric indications has a checkered past because of the profligate use of frontal lobotomy in the mid-twentieth century. This procedure often was used for almost any indication, and the technique was indiscriminant in regards to lesion territory. As a result, many patients who underwent frontal lobotomy suffered severe adverse events, the most common being frontal lobe symptoms such as apathy. In the 1960s, however, neurosurgeons began to lesion much smaller territories in specific brain regions using craniotomy techniques. The result was procedures associated with a much lower incidence of adverse events. Procedures used today include anterior cingulotomy, subcaudate tractotomy, limbic leucotomy (which is tantamount to the combination of an anterior cingulotomy and subcaudate tractotomy), and anterior capsulotomy. All these procedures are performed using craniotomy techniques, although the anterior capsulotomy can be performed using a gamma knife because of its particularly small lesion volume. These procedures have been found to be efficacious in patients suffering from intractable mood and anxiety disorders with response rates ranging from 35% to 70% over a period of several weeks to several months, depending upon the response criteria [4–8]. Common postoperative discomforts include headache, nausea, and edema, all of which usually are temporary. More serious adverse events, including infection, urinary difficulties, weight gain, seizures, cerebral hemorrhage or infarct, and cognitive deficits, are possible but are relatively infrequent and usually are transient [5,7,9].

VAGUS NERVE STIMULATION

VNS was approved by the US Food and Drug Administration (FDA) in 1997 for treatment-resistant epilepsy. VNS involves surgically placing electrodes around the left vagus nerve (the right vagus nerve is not used because it has parasympathetic branches to the heart), which are attached to an internal pulse generator (IPG) placed subcutaneously in the left subclavicular region. Depending upon how the IPG is programmed, intermittent electrical charges of varying magnitude, duration, and frequency can be delivered to the left vagus nerve. Because 80% of the fibers in the vagus nerve are afferent, this electrical charge is predominantly sent to the brain. The left vagus nerve innervates the nucleus tractus solitarius. The nucleus tractus solitarius then communicates with the parabrachial nucleus, the cerebellum, the raphe, the periaqueductal gray, the locus coeruleus, and ascending projections to limbic, paralimbic, and cortical regions. The parabrachial nucleus communicates with the hypothalamus, thalamus, amygdala, and nucleus of the stria terminalis. Of course, the thalamus has projections to the insula, oribitofrontal cortex, and prefrontal cortices; the locus coeruleus and raphe nuclei contain the cell bodies of noradrenergic and serotonergic neurons that then project throughout the central nervous system [10].

Over the course of using VNS to treat more than 40,000 patients who had treatment-resistant epilepsy, it was noted that many of these patients experienced improvement in mood [11,12]. Therefore, trials of VNS for TRD were conducted, and the FDA approved VNS approved for TRD in 2005. The first of these clinical trials assessed adjunctive VNS therapy to sham treatment in patients who had TRD. All patients continued to receive treatment as usual (TAU) in addition to active VNS or sham VNS treatment. There were 112 patients in the active VNS treatment group, and 110 patients received sham VNS treatment for 8 weeks. In this short-term study, VNS therapy failed to exhibit statistically significant efficacy on the primary outcome measure [13]. Patients in both groups (a total of 205 patients) went on to receive open active adjunctive treatment with VNS therapy for 1 year. At 1 year, 27.2% of patients responded, and 15.8% met criteria for remission. In addition, the rates of response and remission doubled from 3 months to 12 months, suggesting that longer-term treatment may be required with VNS [14]. Last, the patients who had TRD receiving adjunctive VNS therapy during the 1-year follow-up study were compared with a matched group of 124 patients who had TRD and who received only TAU. The difference in response rates with VNS plus TAU (19.6%) versus TAU only (12.1%) was not statistically significant. There was, however, a statistically significant difference between remission rates with VNS therapy plus TAU (13.2%) and TAU alone (3.2%) [15]. The data from these clinical trials resulted in FDA approval of VNS for TRD in 2005.

The surgical procedure for placement of the VNS device includes an incision on the left neck so the vagus nerve can be accessed through the carotid sheath and an incision on the left chest in the subclavicular region so the IPG can be implanted. In addition to the potential risks associated with the surgical procedure, a number of side effects were associated with VNS stimulation [14]. The most common was voice alteration (54%–60% of patients) because of the stimulation of the laryngeal and pharyngeal branches of the vagus nerve. Other side effects included cough, neck pain, paresthesia, and dyspnea. The VNS device typically is programmed to deliver intermittent electrical stimulation to the vagus nerve for 30 seconds duration every 5 minutes. The majority of patients treated with VNS experience side effects during the 30-second stimulation period. If patients wish to turn the device off temporarily, they can place a magnet provided by the manufacturer over the IPG. When the magnet is removed, the IPG returns to its previously determined stimulation parameters. Last, rates of worsening depression during the 12-month trial varied from 4% to 7%, seven patients attempted suicide, and three patients became manic [14]. Twenty-four of the clinical trial patients who had TRD receiving VNS discontinued treatment. Seven discontinued because of adverse events, and 17 discontinued because of lack of efficacy.

In summary, VNS seems to be a welcome addition to the available treatments for TRD. The clinical trial data suggest that VNS plus TAU is more efficacious than TAU alone. In addition, the side effects typically are tolerable: only 7 of the 205 patients in the 1-year clinical trial discontinued because of adverse events. The FDA approval states that VNS is an adjunctive treatment for TRD and that it should be used in patients who have severe, chronic, recurrent TRD who have not responded to at least four adequate antidepressant trials.

TRANSCRANIAL MAGNETIC STIMULATION

Repetitive transcranial magnetic stimulation (rTMS) uses a strong magnetic field introduced on the scalp surface to generate focal electrical stimulation of the cortical surface. This focal stimulation, which does not result in a seizure or require anesthesia, is in contrast to the global stimulation resulting in a seizure required for ECT. Potential benefits of rTMS include the ability to administer treatment in an office setting without the use of anesthesia and the possibility of efficacious treatment of major depressive disorder without the cognitive side effects that may occur after treatment with ECT.

There have been a large number of clinical trials of rTMS for major depressive disorder. Most, however, involved small sample sizes, and there was considerable variability in the target area for stimulation and the stimulation parameters. Therefore, meta-analyses, despite their limitations, are informative regarding the efficacy of rTMS for depression. Most included only studies in which the left dorsolateral prefrontal cortex was the stimulation site, and most included only controlled trials. Of the seven published meta-analyses [16–22], six found that rTMS was effective for treating depression. In summary, most found that active rTMS treatment was associated with better outcome than sham control. Most studies were 2 weeks long, although the few longer studies have suggested that the longer course may be associated with better outcome. Also, the majority of studies used high-frequency stimulation to the left dorsolateral prefrontal cortex, although some studies of low-frequency stimulation to the right dorsolateral prefrontal cortex have demonstrated efficacy.

Recently, the results of a large, 23-site study of 6 weeks' duration of active high-frequency rTMS over the left dorsolateral cortex compared with sham

TMS treatment were presented [23]. This trial included 301 patients who had depression and who had not received benefit from at least one but no more than four antidepressant treatments during their current episode. Active TMS showed significant benefit over sham TMS at 4 weeks and 6 weeks on the primary outcome measures. In addition, response rates ranged from 18.1% to 20.6% for active TMS compared with 11.0% to 11.6% for sham TMS at 4 weeks and 23.9% to 24.5% for active TMS compared with 12.3% to 15.1% for sham TMS at 6 weeks. Patients crossing from prior treatment with sham TMS exhibited response rates of 42% to 44% after 6 weeks of active TMS. Last, the rates of discontinuation rates caused by adverse events were similar in the active and sham TMS group, less than 5%. This study is important because it is the largest rTMS study ever conducted by a large margin, it involved multiple sites, it used a blinded design, and it was of 6 weeks' duration. The results of this study are comparable to other smaller clinical trails of rTMS in that, although active rTMS is statistically superior to sham rTMS, the clinical efficacy is not large. Nonetheless, these data may result in future FDA approval of rTMS for depression (it is approved already in Canada and Israel). Again, given the limited number of treatments available for depression and the prevalence of TRD, any such addition probably would be welcome to practitioners. Nonetheless, to date in the United States, this procedure remains experimental, not approved for general clinical use with regard to this indication.

DEEP BRAIN STIMULATION

DBS involves the placement of electrodes in specified brain regions so that electrical stimulation can be delivered in a targeted manner. The electrodes are attached to subcutaneous IPGs on the chest wall that provide power for the electrical stimulation and allow adjustment of stimulation parameters. DBS in the subthalamic nucleus has been used since 1987 for Parkinson's disease [24]. To date more than 35,000 patients who have Parkinson's disease have been implanted, with the majority receiving benefit [25].

To date, one clinical trial of DBS for depression has been published [26]. DBS electrodes were placed in the subgenual cingulate cortex (approximately Brodmann area 25) bilaterally in six patients who had TRD. At 6 months, four of the six patients were classified as responders. DBS in the anterior limb of the internal capsule has also been studied for intractable obsessive-compulsive disorder and shows promise for this indication as well [27]. Depressive symptoms also improved in the cohort of patients who had obsessive-compulsive disorder undergoing DBS. Clinical trials of DBS in the anterior limb of the internal capsule for major depression are currently underway. To date, this procedure remains an experimental, not approved for general clinical use for this indication.

SUMMARY

This brief review provides an overview of neurotherapeutic interventions for major depression that are available currently or are being studied in clinical trials. The growing utility of surgical and device-related treatments for psychiatric conditions may represent a sea change in the field of psychiatry comparable to that seen in other clinical disciplines. For example, for many years the overwhelming majority of cardiac conditions were treated with medications and behavioral interventions. With the advent of cardiac surgical procedures such as ablation and cardiac bypass surgery and the use of devices such as cardiac stents and pacemakers, the ability to treat cardiac disease has improved dramatically. The hope is that the use of neurotherapeutic interventions will lead to a similar improvement in the treatment of psychiatric illness.

The future of neurotherapeutic interventions in psychiatry may include the use of neuroimaging technology to predict which patients may respond to which procedures (for examples, see Refs. [28,29]) or to guide the placement of DBS electrodes on an individual basis. DBS electrodes also could be placed in multiple brain regions. Clinical trials of cortical stimulation using surgically implanted electrodes on the brain surface are underway. These cortical-surface electrodes could provide cortical stimulation comparable to that induced by rTMS at the same location, obviating the need for visits to a physician for rTMS treatments and providing cortical stimulation of a greater magnitude and for an extended duration. Also, one can foresee surgical interventions in which neurotransmitter release is potentiated either by stimulating appropriate nuclei in the brain or by releasing neurotransmitters or neurotransmitter precursors into target brain regions using cannulae or an implanted device. Neurotrophic factors also could be introduced into target brain regions using analogous techniques. Although the future of neurotherapeutic interventions in psychiatry is hard to predict, it is clear that these treatments will have a growing role in the field.

References

[1] Rush AJ, Trivedi MH, Wisniewski SR, et al. Acute and longer-term outcomes in depressed outpatients requiring one or several treatment steps: a STAR*D report. Am J Psychiatry 2006;163:1905–17.
[2] The UK ECT Review Group. Efficacy and safety of electroconvulsive therapy in depressive disorders: a systematic review and meta-analysis. Lancet 2003;361:799–808.
[3] Rasmussen KG, Sampson SM, Rummans TA. Electroconvulsive therapy and newer modalities for the treatment of medication-refractory mental illness. Mayo Clin Proc 2002;77:552–6.
[4] Dalgleish T, Yiend J, Bramham J, et al. Neuropsychological processing associated with recovery from depression after stereotactic subcaudate tractotomy. Am J Psychiatry 2004;161:1913–6.
[5] Dougherty DD, Baer L, Cosgrove GR, et al. Prospective long-term follow-up of 44 patients who received cingulotomy for treatment-refractory obsessive-compulsive disorder. Am J Psychiatry 2002;159:269–75.
[6] Cosgrove GR, Rauch SL. Stereotactic cingulotomy. Neurosurg Clin N Am 2003;14:225–35.
[7] Greenberg BD, Price LH, Rauch SL, et al. Neurosurgery for intractable obsessive-compulsive disorder and depression: critical issues. Neurosurg Clin N Am 2003;14:199–212.
[8] Montoya A, Weiss AP, Price BH, et al. Magnetic resonance imaging-guided stereotactic limbic leucotomy for treatment of intractable psychiatric disease. Neurosurgery 2002;50:1043–9.

[9] Persaud R, Crossley D, Freeman C. Should neurosurgery for mental disorder be allowed to die out? For & against. Br J Psychiatry 2003;183:195–6.

[10] Nemeroff CB, Mayberg HS, Krahl SE, et al. VNS therapy in treatment-resistant depression: clinical evidence and putative neurobiological mechanisms. Neuropsychopharmacology 2006;31:1345–55.

[11] Elger G, Hoppe C, Falkai P, et al. Vagus nerve stimulation is associated with mood improvements in epilepsy patients. Epilepsy Res 2000;42:203–10.

[12] Harden CL, Pulver MC, Ravdin LD, et al. A pilot study of mood in epilepsy patients treated with vagus nerve stimulation. Epilepsy Behav 2000;1:93–9.

[13] Rush AJ, Marangell LB, Sackeim HA, et al. Vagus nerve stimulation for treatment-resistant depression: a randomized, controlled acute phase trial. Biol Psychiatry 2005;58:347–54.

[14] Rush AJ, Sackeim HA, Marangell LB, et al. Effects of 12 months of vagus nerve stimulation in treatment-resistant depression: a naturalistic study. Biol Psychiatry 2005;58:355–63.

[15] George MS, Rush AJ, Marangell LB, et al. A one-year comparison of vagus nerve stimulation with treatment as usual for treatment-resistant depression. Biol Psychiatry 2005;58: 364–73.

[16] Aare T, Dahl AA, Johansen JB, et al. Efficacy of repetitive transcranial magnetic stimulation in depression: a review of the evidence. Nord J Psychiatry 2003;57:227–32.

[17] Burt T, Lisanby H, Sackeim H. Neuropsychiatric applications of transcranial magnetic stimulation: a meta-analysis. Int J Neuropsychopharmacol 2002;5:73–103.

[18] Couturier JL. Efficacy of rapid-rate repetitive transcranial magnetic stimulation in the treatment of depression: a systematic review and meta-analysis. J Psychiatry Neurosci 2005; 30:83–90.

[19] Holtzheimer PE, Russo J, Avery DH. A meta-analysis of repetitive transcranial stimulation in the treatment of depression. Psychopharmacol Bull 2001;35:149–69.

[20] Kozel F, George MS. Meta-analysis of left prefrontal repetitive transcranial magnetic stimulation (rTMS) to treat depression. J Psychiatr Pract 2002;8:270–5.

[21] Martin JLR, Barbanoj-Rodriguez M, Schlaepfer T, et al. Transcranial magnetic stimulation for treating depression. Br J Psychiatry 2003;182:480–91.

[22] McNamara B, Ray JL, Arthurs OJ, et al. Transcranial magnetic stimulation for depression and other psychiatric disorders. Psychol Med 2001;31:1141–6.

[23] Aaronson S, Avery D, Canterbury R, et al. Transcranial magnetic stimulation: effectiveness and safety in a randomized, controlled, multisite clinical trial and an open-label extension study. Presented at the 45th annual meeting of the American College of Neuropsychopharmacology. Hollywood (FL), December 3–7, 2006.

[24] Benabid AL, Pollack P, Louvineau A, et al. Combined (thalamotomy and stimulation) stereotactic surgery of the VIM thalamic nucleus for bilateral Parkinson's disease. Appl Neurophysiol 1987;50:344–6.

[25] Krack P, Batir A, Van Blercom N, et al. Five-year follow-up of bilateral stimulation of the subthalamic nucleus in advanced Parkinson's disease. N Engl J Med 2003;349:1925–34.

[26] Mayberg HS, Lozano AM, Voon V, et al. Deep brain stimulation for treatment-resistant depression. Neuron 2005;45:651–60.

[27] Greenberg BD, Malone DA, Friehs GM, et al. Three-year outcomes in deep brain stimulation for highly resistant obsessive-compulsive disorder. Neuropsychopharmacology 2006;31: 2384–93.

[28] Rauch SL, Dougherty DD, Cosgrove GR, et al. Cerebral metabolic correlates as potential predictors of response to anterior cingulotomy for obsessive compulsive disorder. Biol Psychiatry 2001;50:659–67.

[29] Dougherty DD, Weiss AP, Cosgrove GR, et al. Cerebral metabolic correlates as potential predictors of response to anterior cingulotomy for treatment of major depression. J Neurosurg 2003;99:1010–7.

Cognitive and Behavioral Therapies for Depression: Overview, New Directions, and Practical Recommendations for Dissemination

Greg Feldman, PhD[a,b,*]

[a]Simmons College, Department of Psychology, 300 the Fenway, Boston, MA 02115, USA
[b]Depression Clinical and Research Program, Massachusetts General Hospital,
50 Staniford Suite 401, Boston, MA 02114, USA

C ognitive-behavioral therapy (CBT) is an efficacious first-line treatment for depression [1], even for patients who present with moderate-to-severe symptoms [2,3]. The goal of this review is to present an overview of the family of psychosocial interventions for depression that are collectively referred to as "CBT." Throughout this review, the term "CT" is used when discussing results of specific studies that employed cognitive therapy as described by A.T. Beck and colleagues [4] or J.S. Beck [5]. Elsewhere, the more generic term "CBT" is used to describe the family of interventions using cognitive and behavioral strategies.

First, a brief history of the development and application of CBT to depression is presented. Next, the techniques traditionally used in CBT are described, and newer techniques and recent augmentations to CBT for depression are discussed. The article then reviews empirical studies addressing two crucial questions. First, how does CBT compare with antidepressant medication in terms of efficacy? Second, given the highly recurrent nature of depression [6], how can CBT help prevent relapse? The article concludes with a discussion of the challenge of disseminating CBT and practical recommendations for integrating CBT for depression into psychiatric treatment.

HISTORY OF COGNITIVE-BEHAVIORAL THERAPY FOR DEPRESSION

CBT for depression reflects a family of interventions targeting, to varying degrees, maladaptive thinking (eg, self-criticism, hopelessness) and behavioral patterns (eg, inactivity, social withdrawal, avoidance). Many intervention packages include techniques to address both cognitions and behavior; some

*Simmons College Department of Psychology, 300 the Fenway, Boston, MA 02115.
E-mail address: greg.feldman@simmons.edu

0193-953X/07/$ – see front matter
doi:10.1016/j.psc.2006.12.001

others are purely behavioral in nature [7]. The most widely studied is CT for depression, developed in the early 1960s by psychiatrist A.T. Beck [4], who had trained as a psychoanalyst. He developed the cognitive model of depression after conducting observational clinical research that examined and ultimately failed to support the psychoanalytic model of depression as anger-turned-inward [8]. Instead, he noted that depressed individuals hold negative mental representations of themselves, their world, and their future. These views are activated by negative life events, leading to negatively-biased information processing. Recently, Beck's innovations in the assessment and treatment of psychiatric disorders, particularly depression, were honored with the prestigious Lasker Award for Clinical Medicine Research.

Behavioral interventions are included to varying degrees in different forms of CBT. CT contains both cognitive and behavioral intervention strategies. Roughly concurrent with the development of CT, primarily or exclusively behavioral interventions for depression were being developed and tested. Some of these interventions evolved, often incorporating cognitive interventions along the way [7,9], to yield several empirically supported interventions including the psychoeducational Coping With Depression course [10], self-control therapy [11], problem-solving therapy [12], and behavioral marital therapy [13,14]. Many of these interventions are limited in that they had been tested primarily in populations exhibiting mild depression and generally have garnered less interest than CT in clinical practice [7]. Recent research discussed later in this review has reawakened interest in purely behavioral therapies, however [15]. For instance, behavioral-activation therapy was recently found to be superior to CT in treating more severe depression [16].

DESCRIPTION OF COGNITIVE-BEHAVIORAL THERAPY INTERVENTIONS

A casual follower of recent randomized controlled trials of CBT for depression can be excused for experiencing some confusion as to what exactly CBT for depression entails. Some recent high-profile studies have applied the full protocol of Beckian CT [2]. Other studies have highlighted components contained within Beckian CT for depression, such as problem-solving techniques [17,18] or behavioral activation [16], whereas others have expanded CT to include novel techniques such as mindfulness meditation [19]. This discussion describes the core CBT techniques targeting maladaptive cognition and behavioral patterns associated with depression and then reviews some recent adaptations and innovations.

In contrast to traditional psychoanalytic therapy, CT for depression is a structured, collaborative, short-term, and problem-focused approach to psychotherapy that involves teaching patients a variety of cognitive and behavioral skills that can be used to combat depression. Treatment typically lasts between 10 and 20 sessions [8], with patients often experiencing considerable symptom reduction after four to six weeks of treatment [20,21].

For cognitively-focused interventions, patients initially are taught to monitor and record negative thoughts (eg, "I am so incompetent, I am sure I will get fired from my job soon") and identify how these thoughts influence unpleasant feelings and somatic sensations as well as maladaptive behaviors. Next, patients are taught to evaluate the accuracy and utility of such thoughts, test them empirically, and generate more adaptive, balanced cognitions (eg, "There are many things I do well at work. This one setback will not be the end of my career"). In addition to learning to modify such day-to-day depressogenic cognitions referred to as "automatic thoughts," patients also are guided through identifying and modifying underlying maladaptive beliefs and assumptions (eg, "If I can't do everything perfectly, no one will like me") and self-schemata (eg, "I am a worthless").

Beckian CT also can include behaviorally oriented interventions called "behavioral activation" to target inertia and increase contact with rewarding experiences. As noted previously, some behaviorally-oriented interventions tend to emphasize these techniques to a greater extent. These techniques can include teaching adaptive problem-solving skills (eg, breaking down overwhelming tasks into smaller goals, weighing pros and cons to help make decisions). Developing such problem-solving skills has been the primary focus of several recent CBT interventions in primary care settings [17,18]. Interventions can be used to increase exposure to experiences that produce feelings of pleasure or mastery. First, a patient may be asked to monitor his or her current activity level and then gradually begin scheduling pleasant events and tackling a series of progressively more challenging goals. More recently, studies have found that behavioral activation as a stand-alone intervention performs equally as well as [15,22] and, in some cases, better than [16] Beckian CT, which includes both behavioral activation and cognitive techniques.

Traditional CBT recently has been augmented with novel techniques designed to promote psychological well-being and to target cognitive reactivity (ie, the tendency to respond to sad moods with increased negative thinking) and impairments in interpersonal functioning. These modified approaches have received empirical support that is reviewed in later sections of this article. Two approaches, well-being therapy and mindfulness-based CT, have been applied as relapse-prevention strategies. Well-being therapy [23] is modeled on theoretical work by Ryff [24] emphasizing that the promotion of mental health requires more than ameliorating mental illness. Well-being therapy applies CBT to help patients become more aware of periods of well-being, however fleeting, and challenge automatic thoughts and behaviors that interrupt such periods of pleasant emotions, making it an emotion-regulation strategy that may be particularly relevant to depression [23,25]. Mindfulness-based cognitive therapy (MBCT) [26] is an eight-week group treatment designed to target cognitive reactivity. MBCT encourages patients to become more objective observers of thoughts and feelings through a blend of CT approaches and training in mindfulness techniques including meditation [27]. The goal of these interventions is to teach patients to take a "decentered" view of their depressogenic thoughts, seeing them as mental events rather than accurate reflections of reality or core aspects of their identity.

The cognitive-behavioral analysis system of psychotherapy (CBASP) [28] is designed for acute treatment of chronic depression by targeting problematic interpersonal patterns through situational analysis (a multistep process with some similarity to the CBT methods for recording and challenging maladaptive thought processes). Unlike traditional CBT, the therapeutic relationship itself is conceptualized as an important agent of change. For instance, therapists are encouraged to discuss the patient's transference reactions [28]. This integration of concepts typically associated with psychodynamic therapy into CBT reflects an intriguing synthesis; however, the highly structured, short-term focus of CBASP is a far cry from traditional psychoanalytic therapy.

HOW DOES COGNITIVE-BEHAVIOR THERAPY COMPARE WITH ANTIDEPRESSANT MEDICATION?

A widely cited meta-analysis has shown a slight advantage for CT over medication in treating depression [1]; however, methodologic limitations in some of these older studies may have favored CT [29]. The National Institute of Mental Health's large-scale, multisite Treatment of Depression Collaborative Research Program (TDCRP) [30] remains an influential study examining the relative advantages of CT and pharmacotherapy (in this case, imipramine). Across all patients, CT and medication showed comparable effects; however, among patients who had severe major depressive disorder, imipramine was found to be superior to CT, which performed comparably to an enhanced placebo at posttreatment evaluation [31]. This latter finding has been influential in guiding treatment recommendations that pharmacotherapy be the first-line approach to treating more severe depression [32].

The methods of the TDCRP have been criticized as not providing a fair test of CT [33] and recent research suggests CT and medication are comparable in treating severe depression. A mega-analysis of more severely depressed patients across four large trials including the TDCRP found no advantage for medication over CT [2]. In a more recent study by DeRubeis and colleagues [3] comparing a 16-week treatment of CT with paroxetine for the treatment of moderate-to-severe major depressive disorder, CT and medication were equally effective after 16 weeks of treatment. Both the TDCRP and this newer study found different levels of relative efficacy of CT versus medication across sites, suggesting the quality of CT is an important variable in clinical trials and may vary across settings [3]. Behavioral-activation therapy also has been demonstrated to perform as well as medication (paroxetine) in patients who have severe depression [16].

Although acute outcomes of CT and medication may be largely comparable, CT has been shown consistently to protect better against relapse. Relapse rates for CBT (26%–30%) are superior to those obtained with medication (60%–64%) according to two meta-analyses [1,34]. In the one-year follow-up analysis of DeRubeis and colleagues' [3] trial, Hollon and colleagues [35] reported that patients who completed 16 weeks of CT with up to three optional booster sessions were much less likely to relapse than patients switched to placebo after 16 weeks (31% versus 76%). At a one-year follow-up, relapse rates for CT were comparable with those of individuals maintained on medication for the year (47.2%).

Combining antidepressants and CBT generally yields only a small advantage [36,37] but may be especially advantageous in more chronic forms of depression where large effects of combining CBT and medication are observed over CBT or medication alone [38,39]. A recent large, multisite study [40] using CBASP [28] to treat chronic depression found considerable advantage for combined treatments over either monotherapy (CBASP or nefazodone). The lack of a CBASP-plus-placebo condition in this study makes it difficult to parse a true drug effect in the combined-treatment condition. Secondary analyses have revealed that the subsample of patients who had a history of childhood trauma (loss of parents at an early age, physical or sexual abuse, or neglect) responded better to CBASP (alone or in combination) than to monotherapy medication [41].

CBT has been identified as a promising nonpharmacologic strategy for treating depression in patients who are unresponsive to a first course of antidepressant medication [42]. A noteworthy finding from the final report of the Sequenced Treatment Alternatives to Relieve Depression (STAR*D) study is the relatively high remission rate (41.9%) among a sample of individuals (n = 61) who received CT after not responding to and discontinuing an initial trial of psychopharmacology (citalopram) [43]. There are important caveats to this finding that do not permit direct comparisons with pharmacologic interventions also offered as a second treatment option in this study [44]. Nonetheless, this finding suggests that switching to CT may be a helpful treatment approach.

In summary, CBT may be comparable to medication for acute treatment yet provide more durable benefits. CBT also has added benefits of being more cost effective than medication in the long term [45] and a more tolerable form of treatment in terms of side effects. Combining treatments may be most effective in chronic depression.

CAN COGNITIVE-BEHAVIORAL THERAPY PREVENT RELAPSE?

As noted previously, CBT for depression seems to prevent relapse better than the acute administration of pharmacotherapy. Some studies have examined the efficacy of CBT and its variants administered after patients have recovered or partially recovered from an episode of depression. In one study, patients who responded to pharmacotherapy were randomized to clinical management or to CBT enhanced with well-being therapy and interventions targeting lifestyle modification [46]. The CBT group had a significantly lower relapse rate at a six-year follow-up. In a separate study of partial responders to pharmacotherapy, CBT was effective in preventing relapse [47]. Another promising relapse-prevention study [19] included patients who had recovered from depression and were randomized to either clinical management or MBCT. MBCT was effective in preventing relapse among patients who had had three or more previous episodes of depression, a finding that recently has been replicated [48].

Is there something unique about CBT as an intervention that helps to protect against relapse? The proposed theoretical mechanism of CT is modification of negative thinking [4]. Reduction in self-reported negative cognition does occur after CBT treatment; however, this change is not specific to CBT and has been found in behavioral-activation treatment [15] and pharmacotherapy [49], neither of which directly targets negative cognition.

Although CBT may not uniquely alter cognitive content, it may have a unique effect on cognitive reactivity, the ease or degree to which negative thoughts are automatically triggered in response to transient sad moods or other depression symptoms. In one study, individuals successfully treated with CBT or pharmacotherapy were asked to complete a self-report measure of negative cognition before and after an experimentally-induced negative mood to measure cognitive reactivity [50]. The CBT group showed much less cognitive reactivity than the pharmacotherapy group, a finding that recently was replicated in a large, randomized, controlled trial [51]. Similarly, there is evidence that, compared with pharmacotherapy or family therapy, CBT may uniquely "unlink" negative cognition from depression symptoms [52]. The degree of cognitive reactivity has been shown to predict subsequent relapse [50,51], suggesting a possible explanation for the durability of the effects of CBT compared with other treatment approaches. CBT may uniquely help stop the downward spiral of negative thinking triggered by negative emotional states, leaving patients less vulnerable to relapse.

THE CHALLENGES OF DISSEMINATION AND PRACTICAL RECOMMENDATIONS FOR TREATMENT DELIVERY

Despite the considerable empirical support for CBT interventions for depression, most patients have very limited access to the types of high-quality, structured CBT interventions delivered in research protocols [7,8]. This is due in part to limited CBT training in more practice-oriented graduate programs and the eclectic orientation of many practitioners. Recent graduates of mental health training programs likely will have had at least limited exposure to CBT during their training. A recent large-scale survey of training directors at accredited psychiatry (MD), psychology (PhD, PsyD), and social work (MSW) training programs found that didactic training in CBT is offered in nearly all training programs (93%–100%) and is required in most (80%–99%) [53]. Supervision in CBT, however, is most widely available in PhD and MD programs and is more likely to be required in MD programs. Of the four groups, PhD programs are most likely to endorse the virtues of evidence-based psychotherapies such as CBT. The encouraging news is that, particularly in MD and PhD training programs, students likely are being exposed to the use CBT to treat depression and are being educated about its merits. Unfortunately, the programs that produce the largest number of graduates and place the greatest emphasis on clinical practice (PsyD and MSW) tend not to require training in CBT.

Many clinicians claim to integrate CBT techniques in their practice, yet it is difficult to know how these techniques are being applied. A survey of 470 practicing psychologists reveals that 89% report using cognitive-behavioral techniques in their practice [54]. As many as 52% of the sample, however, report also using psychodynamic/analytic approaches, which have considerably less empirical support. How can a clinician have confidence that a referral to a mental health professional will result in the patient's receiving high-quality CBT? Here are some questions a provider or patient can ask to learn more about whether a psychotherapist is delivering high-quality CBT.

Does the therapist self-identify as having a CBT orientation, and what is his or her opinion about empirically supported treatments? Insurance company listings often allow or require psychotherapists to indicate orientation and specialties. A therapist may indicate using CBT but actually do so in the context of an eclectic approach blending CBT techniques with approaches that have little or no empiric support. Therapists who hold a dismissive attitude toward empirically supported treatments are unlikely to be invested in providing high-quality CBT.

Is the therapist listed in referral services maintained by organizations committed to the study and dissemination of CBT? The Association for Behavioral and Cognitive Therapies is an organization of scientists and clinicians committed to developing, testing, and disseminating empirically supported psychotherapies including CBT. The Academy of Cognitive Therapy is a nonprofit organization founded by A.T. Beck and leading cognitive therapists and researchers that identifies and certifies clinicians who are qualified and effective cognitive therapists. Online referral services are maintained by both the Association for Behavioral and Cognitive Therapies [55] and Academy of Cognitive Therapy [56].

How closely are symptoms tracked during the course of treatment? Frequent monitoring of symptom severity with psychometrically sound instruments such as the Beck Depression Inventory [57] is a key component of CBT. Consistent with the collaborative spirit of CBT, the patient and therapist regularly discuss degree of symptom improvement from week to week. Consistent with the empiricism at the core of CBT, tracking symptom change allows the therapist to illustrate for the patient when symptom improvements follow use of CBT skills during the week.

How much CBT experience does the therapist have? As noted previously, past clinical trials have noted variability in the efficacy of CT has been observed across study sites [3,33], a finding that has been attributed to degree of clinician's experience with CT.

How much is homework emphasized during treatment? A key feature of CBT is the assignment of homework in which the patient practices the skills learned in session to modify behaviors and cognitions in daily life to promote generalization of the skills. The value of homework in CT has received empiric support. Patients who complete homework tend to yield more benefit from CBT for depression [58].

It is possible that a referring clinician or patient using these questions to survey available therapists in their geographical region will not be able to find an acceptable candidate. Even if a candidate therapist is identified, a patient may be unable to meet with the CBT therapist (eg, because of difficulty obtaining transportation or poor physical mobility). Because of cultural beliefs, a patient may be uncomfortable with the idea of receiving talk therapy. Ideally, this concern can be addressed with education from the referring physician about the scientific support for CBT, but this impasse may not be resolved easily. Alternatively, the candidate therapist may have a long waitlist, and the patient may wish to seek immediate relief while awaiting the initial appointment. When one or more of these barriers to CBT treatment is present, the following are some additional strategies psychiatrists and physicians who do not have CBT training can follow:

Recommend physical activity. A promising line of work suggests that physical exercise may have comparable efficacy to antidepressant medication [59], and this treatment effect seems to be durable 10 months later, especially for those who continue to exercise [60]. Such an intervention is consistent with the behavioral-activation component of CBT [9,16]. Obtaining compliance with recommendations for physical exercise is challenging with general medical patients and may be especially so with patients who are depressed and experiencing the loss of motivation and energy that characterize the disorder. As such, the clinician may choose to use motivational interviewing techniques [61] to explore with a patient the pros and cons of both beginning exercise and remaining sedentary. These techniques can help identify barriers to change and help patients discover their own motivation to change their behavior. It also may be useful to assist the patient with trouble-shooting strategies to address perceived and practical obstacles to beginning regular exercise.

Recommend empirically supported CBT self-help books and websites. Central to the mission of CBT is that it is a short-term therapy that teaches patients skills ultimately to "be their own therapists" [5]. Taking this idea one step further, there has been increased interest in self-administered CBT for depression. There is evidence that CBT for depression can be delivered effectively through self-help books [62,63]. Two self-help books that provide an introduction to CBT skills, have received empirical support, and are widely available are *Feeling Good* [64] and *Mind Over Mood* [65]. Web-based CBT has received also empirical support [66]. The interactive, Web-based MoodGym program (www.moodgym.com) consists of five interactive modules that teach CBT skills and can be used by patients without charge. This program was found to be effective at reducing symptoms of depression in a randomized, controlled trial [67].

PROMISING FUTURE DIRECTIONS FOR DISSEMINATION

The shortage of high-quality CBT therapists may be addressed in the future by several promising developments. First, as previously noted, the future generation of psychiatrists and doctoral clinical psychologists currently in training are likely to learn CBT for depression in their training programs [53]. Second, recent studies suggest that CBT may be integrated effectively into primary care settings, thus increasing access for patients outside of traditional mental health centers [17,18,68]. For instance, one recent study found empirical support for having masters-level clinicians deliver CBT by telephone to primary care patients starting antidepressant treatment [68]. Third, the discovery that behavioral activation is an essential ingredient in CBT may be especially crucial to widening dissemination. Researchers of behavioral-activation therapy suggest that behavioral activation is a more parsimonious, and thus readily exportable, form of treatment than CT. As such, behavioral activation may one day be delivered effectively by less experienced therapists and paraprofessionals or in the context of peer support groups or self-administered treatments [15,16]. In short, many promising novel strategies for delivering CBT for depression are awaiting widespread implementation.

SUMMARY

CBT for depression consists of a family of empirically supported interventions that teach patients skills to change maladaptive thinking and behavioral patterns. Recently, CBT has been augmented with techniques to increase psychological well-being and decrease cognitive reactivity and interpersonal dysfunction. CBT for depression has been shown to have efficacy comparable to antidepressant medication across several studies, including samples of moderately to severely depressed patients. The treatment recommendation that pharmacotherapy be the first-line approach to treating more severe depression is largely informed by a single study (the Treatment of Depression Collaborative Research Program) and has not been supported in subsequent research. In light of these newer studies, this recommendation has become controversial, and some have called for its revision.

Although acute outcomes of CBT and medication may be largely comparable, CT consistently has been shown to protect better against relapse. Combining CBT and antidepressant medications treatments may be most effective in the treatment of chronic depression. Recent studies have found that CBT may uniquely reduce cognitive reactivity, which has been shown to be a risk factor for relapse in recovered patients. Pharmacotherapy has been shown to be less effective than CBT in addressing this risk factor.

CBT didactics and supervision are being offered increasingly in training programs for mental health providers including psychiatrists, psychologists, and social workers. Clinicians have widely adopted CBT techniques. When seeking a CBT therapist, however, it is important for a referring clinician or patient to assess the degree to which a therapist actually is practicing high-quality CBT. Some guidelines for making this determination were presented in this review. Additional strategies were discussed for integrating CBT into treatment in situations when access to a high-quality CBT therapist is limited. The article concluded with a review of promising new strategies that may ultimately lead to more widespread dissemination of CBT.

Acknowledgments
The author acknowledges the thoughtful comments of Christopher Beevers, PhD, on an earlier draft of this manuscript and Julie Smith for her assistance with the preparation of this manuscript.

References

[1] Gloaguen V, Cottraux J, Cucherat M, et al. A meta-analysis of the effects of cognitive therapy in depressed patients. J Affect Disord 1998;49:59–72.

[2] DeRubeis RJ, Gelfand LA, Tang TZ, et al. Medications versus cognitive behavior therapy for severely depressed outpatients: mega-analysis of four randomized comparisons. Am J Psychiatry 1999;156:1007–13.

[3] DeRubeis RJ, Hollon SD, Amsterdam JD, et al. Cognitive therapy vs. medications in the treatment of moderate to severe depression. Arch Gen Psychiatry 2005;62:409–16.

[4] Beck AT, Rush AJ, Shaw BF, et al. Cognitive therapy of depression. New York: Guilford Press; 1979.

[5] Beck JS. Cognitive therapy: basics and beyond. New York: Guilford Press; 1995.

[6] American Psychiatric Association. Diagnostic and statistical manual of mental disorders, DSM-IV-TR. 4th edition. Washington, DC: American Psychiatric Association; 2000.

[7] Hollon SD, Thase ME, Marcovitz JC. Treatment and prevention of depression. Psychological Science in the Public Interest 2002;3:39–77.

[8] Beck AT. How an anomalous finding led to a new system of psychotherapy. Nat Med 2006;12:8–15.

[9] Hopko DR, Lejuez CW, Ruggiero KJ, et al. Contemporary behavioral activation treatments for depression: procedures, principles, and progress. Clin Psychol Rev 2003;23:699–717.

[10] Lewinsohn PM, Hoberman HM, Clarke GN. The coping with depression course: review and future directions. Canadian Journal of Behavioral Science 1989;21:470–93.

[11] Rehm LP. A self-control model of depression. Behav Ther 1977;8:787–804.

[12] Nezu AM. Cognitive appraisal of problem solving effectiveness: relation to depression and depressive symptoms. J Clin Psychol 1986;42:42–8.

[13] Jacobson NS, Dobson KS, Fruzzetti A, et al. Social-learning based marital therapy as a treatment for depression. J Consult Clin Psychol 1991;59:547–53.

[14] O'Leary KD, Beach SRH. Marital therapy: a viable treatment for depression and marital discord. Am J Psychiatry 1990;147:183–6.

[15] Jacobson NS, Dobson KS, Truax PA, et al. A component analysis of cognitive-behavioral treatment for depression. J Consult Clin Psychol 1996;64:74–80.

[16] Dimidjan S, Hollon D, Dobson KS, et al. Randomized trial of behavioral activation, cognitive therapy, and antidepressant medication in the acute treatment of adults with major depression. J Consult Clin Psychol 2006;74:658–70.

[17] Barrett JE, Williams JW, Oxman TE, et al. Treatment of dysthymia and minor depression in primary care. J Fam Pract 2001;50:405–12.

[18] Unutzer J, Katon W, Callahan C, et al. Collaborative care management of late-life depression in the primary care setting: a randomized controlled trial. JAMA 2002;288:2836–45.

[19] Teasdale JD, Segal ZV, Williams JMG, et al. Prevention of relapse/recurrence in major depression by mindfulness based cognitive therapy. J Consult Clin Psychol 2000;68: 615–23.

[20] Ilardi SS, Craighead WE. The role of nonspecific factors in cognitive-behavior therapy for depression. Clinical Psychology: Science and Practice 1994;1:138–55.

[21] Tang TZ, DeRebeus RJ. Sudden gains and critical sessions in cognitive-behavioral therapy for depression. J Consult Clin Psychol 1999;67:894–904.

[22] Gortner ET, Gollan JK, Dobson KS, et al. Cognitive-behavioral treatment for depression: relapse prevention. J Consult Clin Psychol 1998;66:377–84.

[23] Fava GA. Well-being therapy: conceptual and technical issues. Psychother Psychosom 1999;68:171–9.
[24] Ryff CD. Happiness is everything, or is it? Explorations on the meaning of psychological well-being. J Pers Soc Psychol 1989;57:1069–81.
[25] Feldman G, Joorman J, Johnson S. Responses to positive affect: a self-report measure of rumination and dampening. Cognit Ther Res, in press.
[26] Segal ZV, Williams JMG, Teasdale JD. Mindfulness-based cognitive therapy for depression: a new approach to preventing relapse. New York: Guilford Press; 2002.
[27] Kabat-Zinn J. Full catastrophe living. New York: Bantam Dell; 1990.
[28] McCullough JP. Treatment for chronic depression: cognitive behavioral analysis system of psychotherapy. New York: Guilford Press; 2000.
[29] Butler AC, Chapman JE, Forman EM, et al. The empirical status of cognitive-behavioral therapy: a review of meta-analyses. Clin Psychol Rev 2006;26:17–31.
[30] Elkin I, Shea MT, Watkins JT, et al. National Institute of Mental Health Treatment of Depression Collaborative Research Program: general effectiveness of treatments. Arch Gen Psychiatry 1989;46:971–82.
[31] Elkin I, Gibbons RD, Shea MT, et al. Initial severity and differential treatment outcome in the National Institute of Mental Health Treatment of Depression Collaborative Research Program. J Consult Clin Psychol 1995;63:841–7.
[32] American Psychiatric Association. Practice guidelines for the treatment of patients with major depressive disorder (revision). Am J Psychiatry 2000;157:1–45.
[33] Jacobson NS, Hollon SD. Cognitive-behavior therapy versus pharmacotherapy: now that the jury's returned its verdict, it's time to present the rest of the evidence. J Consult Clin Psychol 1996;64:74–80.
[34] DeRubeis RJ, Crits-Christoph P. Empirically supported individual and group psychological treatments for adult mental disorders. J Consult Clin Psychol 1998;66:37–52.
[35] Hollon SD, DeRubeis RJ, Shelton RC, et al. Prevention of relapse following cognitive therapy vs medications in moderate to severe depression. Arch Gen Psychiatry 2005;62:417–22.
[36] Hollon SD, Beck AT. Cognitive and cognitive behavioral therapies. In: Bergin AE, Garfield SL, editors. Handbook of psychotherapy and behavioral change. New York: John Wiley & Sons Inc; 1994. p. 428–66.
[37] Otto MW, Smits JAJ, Reese HE. Combined psychotherapy and pharmacotherapy for mood and anxiety disorders in adults: review and analysis. Clinical Psychology: Science and Practice 2005;12:72–86.
[38] Blackburn IM, Bishop S, Glen AIM, et al. The efficacy of cognitive therapy in depression: a treatment trial using cognitive therapy and pharmacotherapy, each alone and in combination. Br J Psychiatry 1981;139:181–9.
[39] Bowers WA. Treatment of depressed in-patients: cognitive therapy plus medication, relaxation plus medication, and medication alone. Br J Psychiatry 1990;156:73–8.
[40] Keller MB, McCullough JP, Klein DN, et al. A comparison of nefazodone, the cognitive behavioral-analysis system of psychotherapy, and their combination for the treatment of chronic depression. N Engl J Med 2000;342:1462–70.
[41] Nemeroff CB, Heim CM, Thase ME, et al. Differential responses to psychotherapy versus pharmacotherapy in patients with chronic forms of major depression and childhood trauma. Proc Natl Acad Sci U S A 2003;100:14293–6.
[42] Shelton RC. Management of major depressive disorder following failure of first antidepressant treatment. Prim psychiatry 2006;13:73–82.
[43] Rush AJ, Trivedi MH, Wisniewski SR, et al. Acute and longer-term outcomes in depressed outpatients requiring one or several treatment steps: a STAR*D report. Am J Psychiatry 2006;163:1905–17.
[44] Nelson JC. The STAR*D study: a four-course meal that leaves us wanting more. Am J Psychiatry 2006;163:1864–6.

[45] Antonuccio DO, Thomas M, Danton WG. A cost-effectiveness analysis of cognitive behavior therapy and fluoxetine (Prozac) in the treatment of depression. Behav Ther 1997;28: 187–210.

[46] Fava GA, Ruini C, Rafanelli C, et al. Six-year outcome of cognitive behavior therapy for prevention of recurrent depression. Am J Psychiatry 2004;161:1872–6.

[47] Paykel ES, Scott J, Teasdale JD, et al. Prevention of relapse in residual depression by cognitive therapy. Arch Gen Psychiatry 1999;56:829–35.

[48] Ma SH, Teasdale JD. Mindfulness-based cognitive therapy for depression. J Consult Clin Psychol 2004;72:31–40.

[49] Fava M, Bless E, Otto M, et al. Dysfunctional attitudes in major depression: changes with pharmacotherapy. J Nerv Ment Dis 1994;182:45–9.

[50] Segal ZV, Germar MC, Williams S. Differential cognitive therapy or pharmacotherapy for unipolar depression. J Abnorm Psychol 1999;108:3–10.

[51] Segal ZV, Kennedy S, Gemar M, et al. Cognitive reactivity to sad mood provocation and the prediction of depressive relapse. Arch Gen Psychiatry 2006;63:749–55.

[52] Beevers CG, Miller IW. Unlinking negative cognition and symptoms of depression: evidence of a specific treatment effect for cognitive therapy. J Consult Clin Psychol 2005;73:68–77.

[53] Weissman MM, Verdeli H, Gameroff MJ, et al. National survey of psychotherapy training in psychiatry, psychology, and social work. Arch Gen Psychiatry 2006;63:925–34.

[54] Meyers L. Psychologists and psychotropic medication. Monitor on Psychology 2006;37: 46.

[55] Available at: www.abct.org/public. Date accessed: January 26, 2007.

[56] Available at: www.academyofct.org. Date accessed: January 26, 2007.

[57] Beck AT, Steer RA, Brown GK. Manual for Beck Depression Inventory-II. San Antonio (TX): Psychological Corporation; 1996.

[58] Thase ME, Callan JA. The role of homework in cognitive behavior therapy of depression. J Psychotherapy Integration 2006;16:162–77.

[59] Blumenthal JA, Babybak MA, Moore KA, et al. Effects of exercise training on older patients with major depression. Arch Med Interna 1999;159:2349–56.

[60] Babyak M, Blumenthal JA, Herman S, et al. Exercise treatment for major depression: maintenance of therapeutic benefit at 10 months. Psychosom Med 2000;62:633–8.

[61] Miller WR, Rollnick S. Motivational interviewing: preparing people to change addictive behavior. New York: Guilford Press; 1991.

[62] Den Boer PC, Wiersma D, Van Den Bosch RJ. Why is self-help neglected in the treatment of emotional disorders? A meta-analysis. Psychol Med 2004;34:959–71.

[63] Whitfield GE, Williams CJ, Shapiro DA. Assessing the take up and acceptability of a self-help room used by patients awaiting their initial outpatient appointment. Behavioural and Cognitive Psychotherapy 2001;29:333–43.

[64] Burns DD. Feeling good. New York: New American Library; 1980.

[65] Greenberger D, Padesky CA. Mind over mood: change how you feel by changing the way you think. New York: Guilford Press; 1995.

[66] Andersson G, Bergstrom F, Hollandare P, et al. Internet-based self-help for depression: randomised controlled trial. Br J Psychiatry 2005;187:456–61.

[67] Christensen H, Griffiths KM, Jorm AF. Delivering interventions for depression by using the Internet: randomized controlled trial. BMJ 2004;328:265–9.

[68] Simon GE, Ludman EJ, Tutty S, et al. Telephone psychotherapy and telephone care management for primary care patients starting antidepressant treatment: a randomized controlled trial. JAMA 2004;292:935–42.

Update and Critique of Natural Remedies as Antidepressant Treatments

David Mischoulon, MD, PhD[a,b,*]

[a]Depression Clinical and Research Program, Department of Psychiatry, Massachusetts General Hospital, WAC-812, 15 Parkman Street, Boston, MA 02114, USA
[b]Harvard Medical School, Boston, MA, USA

N atural or "alternative" remedies have been routinely used in Asia and Europe for centuries [1], and the popularity of these medications in the United States and worldwide has accelerated dramatically over the past decade. Increasing numbers of patients now are asking their doctors whether they might benefit from natural treatments, and many patients see a variety of practitioners in addition to physicians, including herbalists, naturopaths, and other healers. Because natural remedies are readily available over the counter, many individuals are choosing to self-medicate without professional supervision.

The National Institutes of Health has recognized that up to 25% of people in the United States seek and obtain alternative treatments [2], and Eisenberg and colleagues [3] found that 33% of patients at Boston's Beth Israel Medical Center use some form of complementary and alternative medicine. In 1990 there were more visits to alternative treatment practitioners nationwide than to primary care physicians [3]. The World Health Organization reported that that more than 70% of the world's population uses nonconventional medicine [4]. Growing numbers of academic investigators are performing clinical and basic research on these agents, and medical schools and residency training programs are starting to include complementary and alternative medicine in their curricula. Most physicians, however, still feel relatively unequipped to advise patients

The author has received research support from the following companies: Schwabe, NordicNaturals, Amarin (Laxdale Ltd), Lichtwer, Cederroth, SwissMedica, and Bristol-Meyers-Squibb. This publication was made possible in part by grant number 5K23AT001129-05 from the National Center for Complementary and Alternative Medicine. Its contents are solely the responsibility of the author and do not necessarily represent the official views of the National Center for Complementary and Alternative Medicine, National Institutes of Health.

*Depression Clinical and Research Program, Department of Psychiatry, Massachusetts General Hospital, WAC-812, 15 Parkman Street, Boston, MA 02114. E-mail address: dmischoulon@partners.org

0193-953X/07/$ – see front matter
doi:10.1016/j.psc.2006.12.003

who ask about alternative treatments, and many practitioners remain highly skeptical of their potential value.

The benefits and liabilities of herbal remedies and other natural treatments still are largely unclear. Medical research has historically overlooked this area, and nutraceutical companies do not routinely fund studies on these medications [5]. Perhaps the most unfortunate—and dangerous—public misconception about these alternative medications is the belief that, just because something is "natural," it is automatically safe. Although historically the relatively few reports of serious adverse effects from these medications have been a large part of their appeal [1], there increasingly have been cases of individuals who have had toxic reactions from these agents, whether or not they exceeded the recommended dosage [1,6]. Likewise, there are limited data regarding the safety and efficacy of combining alternative medications with conventional ones, but reports of adverse interactions have begun to emerge for some substances.

Natural medications, with the exception of homeopathic remedies, generally are not regulated by the US Food and Drug Administration (FDA) [5,7]. Consequently, optimal doses for these medications are poorly established, as are the active ingredients, contraindications, drug–drug interactions, and potential toxicities. Another consequence of the lack of regulation is that preparations made by different companies vary in regard to form, quality, or purity of the medication—and hence in effectiveness.

Although natural medications are available for most physical and medical problems, there are relatively fewer ones for psychiatric disorders, and these treatments are mainly limited to mood and anxiety symptoms and senescent cognitive decline. This article reviews three of the best-studied natural medications for mood disorders, St. John's Wort (hypericum), S-adenosyl methionine (SAMe), and the omega-3 fatty acids eicosapentaenoic acid (EPA) and docosahexaenoic acid (DHA).

ST. JOHN'S WORT

Hypericum is an extract of the flower of St. John's Wort (*Hypericum perforatum L.*) that has been used for the treatment of depression for centuries [1]. Physicians in Europe have long considered hypericum effective for treating mild-to-moderate depression. In the past decade, interest in St. John's Wort has increased dramatically in the United States and worldwide, and today it is one of the biggest-selling natural remedies on the market.

Mechanisms of Action

The mechanism of action of hypericum is not fully understood. The extract from St. John's Wort contains polycyclic phenols, hypericin and pseudohypericin, which are among the presumed active components; other compounds include flavonoids (hyperoside, quercetin, isoquercitrin, rutin), kaempferol, luteolin, biapigenin, and hyperforin [8–10]. Hypericin, believed to be one of the main active components in hypericum, decreases serotonin receptor density

[11]. Because hypericin does not cross the blood–brain barrier, one proposed mechanism of action for hypericin is the inhibition of monocyte cytokine production of interleukin 6 and 1β, resulting in a decrease in corticotropin releasing hormone and thus dampening production of cortisol [12]. Hypericin also may inhibit reuptake of serotonin, norepinephrine, and dopamine [11] and may thus result in reduced expression of beta adrenoreceptors and increased density of serotonin (5-HT_{2A} and 5-HT_{1A}) receptors [13]. Hypericin also may have affinity for γ-aminobutyric acid receptors.

More recent investigations have implicated hyperforin as a possible active ingredient [14]. Laakmann and colleagues [15] performed a randomized, double-blind, placebo-controlled 6-week study of two different extracts of hypericum, on 147 patients. The two extracts contained 0.5% and 5% hyperforin, respectively. Patients who received the hypericum extract with 5% hyperforin showed greater improvement in mean Hamilton Depression Scale (HAM-D) scores than the group receiving the 0.5% hyperforin extract, and the latter group showed only slightly greater improvement than the placebo group.

Various mechanisms of antidepressant action for hyperforin have been proposed, including serotonin reuptake inhibition and norepinephrine and acetylcholine reuptake inhibition. Some studies suggest inhibition of serotonin, dopamine, norepinephrine, γ-aminobutyric acid , and L-glutamate [16], although serotonergic mechanisms probably are most important. Other mechanisms have been proposed also, including reduced expression of cortical beta-adrenoceptors and 5-HT_2 receptors and synaptosomal release similar to that caused by reserpine [14].

Other components of hypericum, including the flavonoids, are irreversible monoamine oxidase-A inhibitors, but the concentration of these compounds in the extract are so small that they are unlikely to be involved in the antidepressant mechanism [17].

Most commercially available St. John's Wort preparations are standardized either to hypericin or hyperforin. Because there are several different preparations of the medication, the amount of other active ingredients may vary with different preparations, and there are no published head-to-head trials with different brands of Hypericum.

Efficacy

In general, hypericum has been reported to have efficacy greater than placebo and equal to active controls. There are approximately 37 published trials, including 26 placebo-controlled studies and 14 with a standard antidepressant as the active comparator [18]. Most studies have been conducted in Europe, usually with patients already in clinical care in general practice settings [1]. Results in such studies may be more predictive of effectiveness and acceptability in clinical practice but may differ widely from results in a controlled research setting. For example, the European studies generally report little about the methods of recruitment, whether consecutive patients were recruited, and what, if any, exclusion criteria were applied. Patient groups in many European studies of hypericum were not limited to major depression and included other diagnoses [1,14].

In clinical trials hypericum has been compared with low doses of both imipramine and maprotiline [19–22]. Doses of imipramine and maprotiline used in European clinical practice tend to be lower than those considered adequate by psychopharmacologists in the United States. In these clinical trials, the typical dose of imipramine or maprotiline is 75 mg/d . Despite the inadequate doses of active controls, the response rates in these trials seemed comparable to those in studies that use higher doses of tricyclic antidepressant agents (TCAs) (eg, imipramine >150 mg/d). The lack of a placebo control makes it difficult to interpret the results, but hypericum seemed to be at least as effective as low doses of imipramine and maprotiline. In these studies, response rates for hypericum ranged from 35.3% to 81.8%, and response for TCAs ranged from 41.2% to 77.8%.

A meta-analysis by Nierenberg [23] examined four studies comprising a heterogeneous group of depressive conditions, in which hypericum, 300 mg three times per day, was judged to be effective in 79 of 120 subjects (65.8%), whereas placebo was considered effective in only 36 of 125 subjects (28.8%; chi square 32.24; $P < .0001$). The placebo response rate seemed comparable to that observed in many outpatient studies of antidepressants conducted in the United States.

A meta-analysis by Linde and colleagues [24] examined 15 trials comparing Hypericum with placebo and eight trials comparing Hypericum with TCAs in 1757 patients who had mild-to-moderate depression. In six trials that used single preparations of Hypericum (containing only St. John's Wort), hypericum yielded greater response rates than placebo (55.1% for Hypericum versus 22.3% for placebo) and comparable response rates to tricyclic antidepressants (63.9% for Hypericum versus 58.5% for tricyclic antidepressants). In two trials that used combination preparations of Hypericum (containing St. John's Wort and other herbal medications such as Kava), Hypericum was found to be more effective than TCAs (67.7% versus 50%). A meta-analysis by Voltz [25] suggested that Hypericum may not be effective for acute treatment of severely depressed patients.

In the last 5 to 6 years, approximately 10 notable studies by North American, European, and South American investigators have been published. Many of these studies are distinguished by their large-scale, randomized, double-blind design and/or by comparing St. John's Wort with newer antidepressants, particularly the selective serotonin reuptake inhibitors (SSRIs), as well as with placebo.

In a 6-week trial with 375 patients, Lecrubier and colleagues [26] found that St. John's Wort, 900 mg/d, was significantly more effective than placebo, especially in patients who had higher baseline HAM-D scores. In an 8-week trial with 200 depressed subjects, Shelton and colleagues [27] found that St. John's Wort, 900 to 1200 mg/d, was no more effective than placebo in the full intent-to-treat analysis, although among completers the remission rates were significantly higher with St. John's Wort than with placebo.

Brenner and colleagues [28] compared St. John's Wort, 900 mg/d, versus sertraline 75, mg/d, in 30 depressed subjects for 6 weeks. St. John's Wort yielded a 47% response rate and sertraline a 40% response rate. The difference was not statistically significant. Gastpar and colleagues [29] also compared St. John's Wort, 612 mg/d, against sertraline, 50 mg/d, in 241 depressed subjects for 12 weeks, with 161 subjects receiving an additional 12 weeks of treatment for a total treatment period of 6 months. By the first 12 weeks, Hypericum was found to yield a response rate comparable to sertraline, and this response was maintained in subjects who continued for the full 6 months. van Gurp and colleagues [30] compared St. John's Wort, 900 to 1800 mg/d, with sertraline, 50 to 100 mg/d, in 12 community-based primary care offices. Eighty-seven depressed subjects were treated for 12 weeks. No significant differences in mean HAM-D scores were found, and St. John's Wort resulted in significantly fewer adverse events.

Schrader [31] compared St. John's Wort, 500 mg/d, with fluoxetine, 20 mg/d, for 6 weeks in 240 depressed subjects. St. John's Wort yielded a 60% response rate and fluoxetine a 40% response rate. Results barely reached significance in favor of St. John's Wort. The authors noted that St. John's Wort had a more favorable adverse-effects profile. Only 8% of subjects receiving St. John's Wort reported adverse events compared with 23% receiving fluoxetine. Behnke and colleagues [32] compared St. John's Wort with fluoxetine in 70 mildly to moderately depressed subjects for 6 weeks. They found HAM-D score decreases of 50% for St. John's Wort and 58% for fluoxetine, with the efficacy of St. John's Wort approximately 80% of that of fluoxetine on the HAM-D and the von Zerssen Depression scales.

The Hypericum Depression Study Group [33] compared St. John's Wort at doses of 900 to 1500 mg/d versus sertraline, 50 to 100 mg/d, or placebo for 8 weeks in 340 depressed subjects. St. John's Wort and sertraline both yielded a response rate of approximately 24%; the response rate for placebo was 32%. This report, along with that of Shelton and colleagues [27], resulted in a great deal of media attention during 2002, and St. John's Wort sales worldwide dropped temporarily in the immediate aftermath [5].

Fava and colleagues [34] at the Massachusetts General Hospital (MGH) conducted a study similar to the Hypericum Group's, comparing St. John's Wort, 900 mg/d, with fluoxetine, 20 mg/d, versus placebo for 12 weeks. The study was powered for 180 subjects, but the sponsor closed the study prematurely because of the media hysteria over the previously mentioned negative studies, which were published while the MGH study was in progress. Consequently, only 135 subjects were recruited. The results showed a trend toward significance for St. John's Wort against placebo with regard to decrease in HAM-D scores and a significant advantage for St. John's Wort against fluoxetine. Remission rates were 38% for St. John's Wort, 30% for fluoxetine, and 21% for placebo, but these differences did not reach significance. In view of the placebo response rate, which was consistent with the literature, the authors concluded that the observed results were "real" and suggested that if the full complement of 180 subjects had been recruited, both St. John's Wort and fluoxetine would have beaten placebo by a statistically significant margin.

Moreno and colleagues [35] compared hypericum, 900 mg/d, with fluoxetine, 20 mg/d, or placebo in 72 depressed subjects. After 8 weeks, the authors found that hypericum yielded a remission rate of 12%, significantly lower than that of fluoxetine (34.6%) and placebo (45%).

How should these recent studies be interpreted in the context of the previous literature? A recent Cochrane review declared similar response rates overall for St. John's Wort, SSRIs, and TCAs but cautioned about the "inconsistent and confusing" nature of the data [18]. In comparisons between St. John's Wort and placebo, the results tended to favor St. John's Wort but more so in cases where there was not a strict diagnosis of major depressive disorder. Trials with strictly diagnosed depression according to *Diagnostic and Statistic Manual of Mental Disorders*, 4th edition (DSM) criteria showed less robust results [18]. More studies are necessary to clarify some of the questions about efficacy that the aforementioned studies have raised.

Safety and Tolerability

In the past few years, increasing numbers of adverse drug–drug interactions between St. John's Wort and other medications have been reported in the literature. These interactions are thought to occur largely through the liver enzyme CYP-450-3A4 and have resulted in decreased activity of several drugs, including warfarin, cyclosporin, oral contraceptives, theophylline, phenprocoumon, digoxin, indinavir, and irinotecan [36–40]. Extreme caution, therefore, is required with HIV-positive patients who take protease inhibitors, cancer patients receiving chemotherapy, and transplant recipients who take immunosuppressive drugs. It also is recommended that St. John's Wort not be combined with SSRIs, because anecdotes of "serotonin syndrome" have been reported, presumably related to St. John's Wort's monoamine oxidase inhibitor activity [41].

When St. John's Wort is used as monotherapy, adverse events are relatively uncommon and mild [42]. Patients have complained of dry mouth, dizziness, constipation, other gastrointestinal symptoms, and confusion [1,42]. Woelk and colleagues [43] followed 3250 patients treated with hypericum by 633 physicians in routine clinical practice and found that only 2.4% of patients mentioned side effects of gastrointestinal symptoms and allergic reactions. Only 1.5% of patients stopped taking the drug because of these side effects. So far, there seem to be no published reports assessing the effects of an hypericum overdose.

Phototoxicity has long been associated with hypericum in grazing animals and has been reported, albeit rarely, in humans [44]. Brockmoller and colleagues [45] found that doses of hypericum as high as 1800 mg caused minor increases in sensitivity to UV light in humans but no phototoxicity. Siegers and colleagues [46] have recommended that patients who take an overdose of hypericum should be isolated from UV radiation for 7 days, but this caution may not necessarily apply to patients receiving regular doses. As a general precaution, the author and colleagues recommend that patients who take St. John's Wort use sunscreen and other protection when spending large amounts of time in the sun.

At least 17 cases of psychosis resulting from St. John's Wort have been reported, of which 12 comprised mania or hypomania [47]. Bipolar patients therefore should be advised to use St. John's Wort only with a concurrent mood stabilizer.

Recommendations

Hypericum has been shown to be more effective than placebo and equal to low-dose TCAs in most controlled trials but has had less impressive results against the SSRIs and placebo in the more recent studies, perhaps in part because of the recruitment of more severely and/or chronically depressed patient samples [14].

Recommended doses of St. John's Wort based on the literature fall between 900 mg and 1800 mg/d, usually divided on a twice- or thrice-daily basis. St. John's Wort seems to have a relatively benign side-effect profile, although, given the risk of interactions, care needs to be taken with patients taking multiple medications. Likewise, in view of the risk of cycling, caution should be exercised in patients who have bipolar disorder.

The literature as a whole suggests that St. John's Wort may be less effective in cases of more severe and/or more chronic depression, and people who have milder forms of depression therefore may be the best candidates for St. John's Wort. A collaborative study of St. John's Wort for minor depression is currently in progress at MGH and Cedars-Sinai Medical Center. Hypericum needs to be studied further in depressed subjects who have rigorously diagnosed DSM-IV major depression, using placebo and active controls for acute treatment periods of at least 8 to 12 weeks. Longer-term continuation treatment also merits investigation, and systematic tracking of side effects needs to be further developed.

S-ADENOSYL METHIONINE

SAMe (Box 1) is a methyl donor in the brain, involved in the pathways for synthesis of hormones, neurotransmitters, nucleic acids, proteins, and phospholipids [48]. Of particular interest is its activity as an intermediate in the synthesis of norepinephrine, dopamine, and serotonin [48], which suggested

---

Box 1: S-adenosyl methionine

$$NH_2\text{-}CH\text{-}CH_2\text{-}CH_2\text{-}S\text{-}Adenosyl$$
$$\quad | \qquad\qquad\qquad |$$
$$O=C\text{-}OH \qquad\quad CH_3$$

This derivative of the amino acid methionine functions by donating a methyl (-CH$_3$) group in a variety of metabolic reactions, including the synthesis of neurotransmitters.

its potential role in mood regulation. Widely prescribed in Europe for decades, SAMe gained popularity in the United States following its release as an over-the-counter dietary supplement in 1998–1999. It is considered a potential treatment for major depression as well as for a number of other medical conditions [48].

Mechanisms of Action

SAMe is synthesized from the amino acid l-methionine through the one-carbon cycle, a metabolic pathway involving the vitamins folate and B_{12} [48]. Deficiencies of both these vitamins have long been associated with depression. For example, 10% to 30% of depressed patients may have low folate, and these patients may respond less well to antidepressants [49]. Administration of folate augmentation to partial responders to antidepressants has yielded encouraging results [50,51]. Vitamin B_{12} is converted to methylcobalamin, which also is involved in the synthesis of various central nervous system neurotransmitters. B_{12} deficiency may result in an earlier age of onset of depression [52]. The final pathway of these vitamin deficiencies may be reduced SAMe, leading to diminished synthesis of vital neurotransmitters. The replenishment of folate and B_{12} may in turn result in increased SAMe and neurotransmitter synthesis. Indeed, low SAMe levels have been found in the cerebrospinal fluid of depressed individuals [53], and higher plasma SAMe levels have been associated with improvement in depressive symptoms [54]. The enzyme methionine adenosine transferase, necessary for the manufacture of SAMe, has decreased activity in depressed schizophrenic patients but increased activity in manic patients [55–57]. If correction of B-vitamin deficiencies can increase SAMe levels and hence alleviate depressive symptoms, it is reasonable to postulate that direct administration of SAMe also could reverse a depressed state.

Efficacy

There are approximately 45 published clinical studies of SAMe for treatment of depression, of which at least 8 are placebo controlled and 8 used an active comparator [48,58–60]. SAMe demonstrated superiority to placebo in six of the eight placebo-controlled studies with sample sizes ranging from 40 to 100 individuals and equivalency to placebo in the other two studies [48,59,60]. In six of eight comparison studies with TCAs, SAMe was equivalent in efficacy to TCAs and was more effective than imipramine in one study [48,59,60]. Doses of SAMe in these studies ranged from 200 to 1600 mg/d administered orally, intramuscularly, or intravenously [48,59,60].

Overall, trials of oral SAMe suggest efficacy comparable to TCAs and superiority to placebo at doses between 200 and 1600 mg/d [48,59,60]. Although some early studies yielded equivocal results because of problems with dissolution and stability of early oral SAMe preparations [48,59,60], current oral SAMe preparations are tosylated and are more stable and thus are more suitable for research use. As yet there are no published reports comparing SAMe against newer antidepressants such as SSRIs, but such studies are in progress.

SAMe may have a relatively faster onset of action than conventional antidepressants [48,59,60]. In one study, some patients improved within a few days, and most did so within 2 weeks [61]. Likewise, two studies showed that the combination of SAMe and a low-dose TCA resulted in earlier onset of action than a TCA alone [62,63].

A recent study by Alpert and colleagues [64] examined the efficacy of SAMe as an adjunctive treatment for partial and nonresponders to SSRIs. Thirty subjects who had residual depression despite SSRI or venlafaxine treatment received a 6-week course of SAMe, 800 to 1600 mg. Response and remission rates with SAMe augmentation were 50% and 43%, respectively, and the treatment was well tolerated. The results suggest a possible role for SAMe as an augmenting agent in cases of partial or nonresponse to SSRIs. As of yet, there are no published studies using a placebo control.

Other reports suggest that SAMe is effective for dementia-related cognitive deficits, depression in patients who have Parkinson's disease or other medical illness, psychologic distress during the puerperium, and opioid and alcohol detoxification [60].

Safety and Tolerability

SAMe is well tolerated and relatively free of adverse effects. There is no apparent hepatotoxicity or anticholinergic effects. Side effects include mild insomnia, lack of appetite, constipation, nausea, dry mouth, sweating, dizziness, and nervousness [48]. Cases of increased anxiety, mania, or hypomania in bipolar depression have been reported [48,65,66], and therefore care must be taken with patients who have a history of bipolar disorder. These patients should be advised not to take SAMe unless they are receiving a concurrent mood stabilizer. So far, there seem to be no significant drug–drug interactions between SAMe and FDA-registered drugs.

Recommendations

There is encouraging evidence that SAMe is effective for treatment of major depression, both as monotherapy and as an adjunct to FDA-approved antidepressants. Some studies have suggested a faster onset of action for SAMe than for conventional antidepressants, and it may accelerate the effect of conventional antidepressants when combined. SAMe seems to be well tolerated, with a relatively benign side-effect profile. It may be especially good for patients who are sensitive to antidepressant-related side effects, particularly the elderly and those who have medical comorbidity. There is no apparent toxicity, except for risk of cycling in patients who have bipolar depression. Recommended doses range from 400 to 1600 mg/d [48,59,60], although in clinical practice the author and colleagues have observed some individuals who require at least 3000 mg/d for alleviation of depression. More research is needed to determine optimal SAMe doses, and head-to-head comparisons with newer antidepressants should help clarify SAMe's place in the psychopharmacologic armamentarium.

SAMe is relatively expensive, with prices ranging from $0.75 to $1.25 for a 400-mg tablet. Because insurance plans do not cover over-the-counter supplements, the out-of-pocket cost can be prohibitive to many patients, particularly those who may require higher doses. Careful shoppers who search the Internet may be able to purchase SAMe at more accessible prices, but they should verify the reputation of the seller. With increasing numbers of manufacturers and competition in the marketplace, it is hoped that the price of SAMe will drop in the foreseeable future.

OMEGA-3 FATTY ACIDS

During the past century, intake of omega-3 fatty acids in the Western diet has decreased dramatically, while intake of processed foods rich in omega-6–containing vegetable oils has increased. This dietary shift has resulted in a higher physiologic ratio of omega-6:omega-3 fatty acids in Western countries compared with countries with higher fish and omega-3 consumption [67–71]. The modern Western diet and the additional stresses of twenty-first century life have been postulated to create a baseline proinflammatory state in humans that may contribute to cardiovascular disease and also may play a role in the development of mood disorders [72]. Administration of omega-3 supplements may potentially reverse this proinflammatory state by correcting the omega-6:omega-3 ratio, thus providing beneficial cardiovascular and mood-related effects. Several recent treatment studies have yielded encouraging, albeit preliminary, evidence of clinical efficacy for omega-3 fatty acids as mood-enhancing agents. The two omega-3 fatty acids thought to be relevant to psychiatry are EPA and DHA (Box 2), both of which are found primarily in fish oil. Investigations into their efficacy have examined EPA and DHA separately and in combination with each other.

Mechanisms of Action

How might the omega-3 fatty acids exert their mood-enhancing effect? Proposed mechanisms for the amelioration of depression include an effect on membrane-bound receptors and enzymes involved in the regulation of

---

Box 2: Docosahexaenoic acid and eicosapentaenoic acid

Docosahexaenoic acid

$CH_3-CH_2-CH=CH-CH_2-CH=CH-CH_2-CH=CH-CH_2-CH=CH-CH_2-CH=CH-CH_2-CH=CH-CH_2-CH_2-COOH$

Docosahexaenoic acid (22:6, n-3) has a 22-carbon chain and six double bonds. The leftmost carbon is termed the "omega" carbon, and the first double bond occurs on the third carbon from the left, hence the term "omega-3."

Eicosapentaenoic acid

$CH_3-CH_2-CH=CH-CH_2-CH=CH-CH_2-CH=CH-CH_2-CH=CH-CH_2-CH=CH-CH_2-CH_2-CH_2-COOH$

Eicosapentaenoic acid (20:5, n-3) has a 20-carbon chain and five double bonds. The first double bond occurs on the third carbon from the left.

neurotransmitter signaling, as well as regulation of calcium ion influx through calcium channels [72]. Hamazaki and colleagues [73] found that administration of a combination of EPA and DHA to healthy subjects resulted in a lowering of plasma norepinephrine levels compared with placebo, and the authors proposed that omega-3s could exert their effect by interaction with the catecholamines. Omega-3 fatty acids also may inhibit secretion of inflammatory cytokines, thus leading to decreased corticosteroid release from the adrenal gland and dampening mood-altering effects associated with cortisol [72,74]. For example, EPA inhibits the synthesis of prostaglandin E2, thus dampening the synthesis of p-glycoprotein, the latter of which may be involved in antidepressant resistance [74]. In this regard, EPA resembles amitriptyline, which also inhibits p-glycoprotein and is generally considered useful for resistant depression.

Efficacy

Approximately half a dozen controlled trials and a few open studies with EPA and/or DHA suggest that supplementation with omega-3 fatty acids at doses about five or more times the standard dietary intake in the United States may yield antidepressant and/or mood stabilizing effects.

Peet and Horrobin [75] conducted a randomized, placebo-controlled, dose-finding study of ethyl-eicosapentaenoate (EPA) as adjunctive therapy for 70 adults who had persistent depression despite treatment with a standard antidepressant. Subjects who received 1 g/d EPA for 12 weeks showed significantly higher response rates (53%) than subjects receiving placebo (29%), with notable improvement of depressed mood, anxiety, sleep disturbance, libido, and suicidality. The 2 g/d group showed little evidence for a drug:placebo difference, and the 4 g/d group showed a nonsignificant trend toward improvement. These results suggest that there may be an optimal dose of omega-3 that humans require for maximum benefit, and it is possible that an overcorrection of the omega-6:omega-3 ratio with higher omega-3 doses may limit the antidepressant effect of EPA.

Su and colleagues [76] conducted an 8-week, double-blind, placebo-controlled trial comparing adjunctive omega-3 (6.6 g/d) against placebo in 28 depressed patients. Patients in the omega-3 group had a significant decrease in HAM-D scores compared with placebo. In a sample of 20 subjects who had major depressive disorder and were receiving antidepressant therapy, Nemets and colleagues [77] found a statistically significant benefit of adjunctive EPA, 1 g/d, and a clinically important difference in the mean reduction of the 24-item HAM-D scale by the study endpoint at week 4 compared with placebo (12.4 versus 1.6). Frangou and colleagues [78] treated 75 depressed subjects with ethyl-EPA at 1 g/d, 2 g/d, or placebo for 12 weeks. EPA outperformed placebo significantly in both EPA treatment arms, based on HAM-D scores; the higher dose of EPA seemed to confer no added benefit compared with 1 g/d.

A recent small study by Silvers [79] suggested that 8 g of "fish oil" was not more effective than 8 g of "olive oil," but this underpowered study was limited by problems with attrition, dosage, and choice of rating scales. Regarding DHA, a single placebo- controlled study with 36 subjects showed lack of efficacy of DHA, 2 g/d, for depression [80].

Freeman and colleagues [81] performed a dose-finding trial of omega-3 in 16 women who had postpartum depression. Subjects received 0.5 g/d, 1.4 g/d, or 2.8 g/d. HAM-D scores and the Edinburgh Post Natal Depression Scale both decreased by approximately 50% for all groups, and there seemed to be no dose–response effect. Marangell and colleagues [82] found no preventive effect of postpartum depression with open omega-3 mix (EPA and DHA), 2960 mg/d, in a small sample of pregnant women.

Omega-3 fatty acids may have efficacy for bipolar as well as unipolar mood disorders. Using high doses of an omega-3 fatty acid mix (6.2 g EPA plus 3.4 g DHA) versus placebo over a 4-month period, Stoll and colleagues [83] found that among 30 patients who had bipolar I or II disorder, a Kaplan-Meier survival analysis revealed a significantly longer duration of remission for those receiving adjunctive omega-3 fatty acid mix versus placebo along with their current mood stabilizing regimen.

Keck and colleagues [84] were unable to replicate Stoll and colleagues' results in a larger-scale study. In their double-blind, placebo-controlled trial of adjunctive EPA, 6 g/d, for 4 months in patients who had bipolar depression (n = 57) or rapid cycling (n = 59), EPA did not separate from placebo. A recent critique of this study suggested that most of the observed benefit in bipolar subjects is with regard to depressive rather than manic symptoms [85].

Osher and colleagues [86] treated 12 bipolar I depressed subjects with open adjunctive EPA, 1.5 to 2 g/d, for up to 6 months. Ten patients completed at least 1 month of follow-up, and eight achieved a 50% or greater reduction in HAM-D scores. No cycling occurred with any patients.

Further investigation is needed to determine whether bipolar disorder actually requires higher doses of omega-3 fatty acids than unipolar illness and to unravel the respective contributions of EPA and DHA.

The relationship between omega-3 fatty acid treatment and a range of other psychiatric syndromes also has been studied to a lesser extent; the resulting data are equivocal. Conditions investigated include borderline personality disorder, schizophrenia, attention-deficit disorder, and obsessive-compulsive disorder [87–94]. These investigations tend to consist of smaller patient samples, and their conflicting results reflect this limitation.

Safety and Tolerability

The omega-3s have been shown to be very safe. Most complaints of side effects such as gastrointestinal upset and fishy aftertaste tend to occur with higher doses (>5 g/d) and with less pure preparations. At the more typical doses of 1 g/d with highly purified omega-3 preparations, these adverse effects are less common. There is a documented risk of bleeding, which seems to be minimal, particularly with doses less than 3 g/d. Individuals taking anticoagulants such as warfarin need to be careful, and should not use omega-3s without physician supervision [95]. Given a few documented cases of cycling in bipolar patients [95], omega-3s should be used with care in this population and preferably with a concomitant mood stabilizer.

Recommendations

The data supporting use of omega-3 fatty acids for depression are encouraging, particularly with regard to EPA. Low doses of omega-3 fatty acids may be effective and well-tolerated monotherapy or adjunctive therapy for depressed adults. A recent review by Freeman and colleagues [95] recommends that depressed individuals may safely use approximately 1 g/d of an EPA-DHA mixture but should not substitute omega-3s for conventional antidepressants at this time. Likewise, individuals who take more than 3 g/d of omega-3 should do so under a physician's supervision [95].

The omega-3 fatty acids may be particularly well suited for treatment of specific patient populations (eg, pregnant or lactating women) for whom antidepressants must be used with caution [96], for elderly people who may not tolerate side effects of conventional antidepressants agents, and for those who have medical comorbidity, particularly cardiovascular disease and possibly autoimmune conditions, for which there may be dual benefits.

Most studies thus far have used omega-3s as adjunctive agents; given their apparent safety and tolerability, their effectiveness as monotherapy should be investigated further. Likewise, the issue of whether EPA or DHA is more effective in the treatment of depression remains to be clarified. Finally, the mechanism of action of the omega-3s, particularly their interplay with the immune system, merits further investigation. Studies addressing these questions are currently underway at the MGH and Cedars-Sinai Medical Center. It is hoped that these and other future investigations will clarify some of the lingering unanswered questions about this exciting and potentially valuable treatment.

SUMMARY

Natural medications such as St. John's Wort, SAMe, and omega-3 fatty acids eventually may prove to be valuable additions to the psychiatrist's pharmacologic armamentarium, both as monotherapy and as adjunctive therapy for mood disorders. Current research data are compelling, from a standpoint of both efficacy and safety, but before clinicians can recommend these as first-line treatments, more well-designed controlled studies in large patient populations are needed. During the past decade, the National Institutes of Health, the National Institute for Mental Health, and the National Center for Complementary and Alternative Medicine have widened their support for research on the efficacy and safety of alternative treatments, and increasing numbers of academic institutions are undertaking large-scale, multicenter studies on the natural medications reviewed here, as well as others. These studies should help answer some of the yet-unsettled questions about natural medications.

Psychiatrists who are considering recommending natural antidepressants to their patients should emphasize that these treatments are relatively unproven and that it remains to be seen whether they would be appropriate or preferable to the conventional psychotropic agents [97,98]. In the absence of more conclusive data, the best candidates for alternative treatments may be patients for whom a delay in adequate treatment would not be devastating (eg, the mildly symptomatic patient who has a strong interest in natural remedies). Other good candidates may include patients who have been unresponsive to conventional antidepressants or particularly intolerant of side effects; these patients, however, often are the most difficult to treat, and alternative agents seem best suited for the mildly ill [98]. Care should be taken with patients who are taking multiple medications, in view of adverse drug–drug interactions that have emerged with increased use of alternative treatments. Finally, as with all psychotropic agents, natural medications should be used preferably under the supervision of a physician.

References

[1] Schulz V, Hansel R, Tyler VE. Rational phytotherapy: a physician's guide to herbal medicine. 4th edition. Berlin: Springer; 2001. p. 78–86.
[2] National Institutes of Health Office of Alternative Medicine 1997. Clinical practice guidelines in complementary and alternative medicine. An analysis of opportunities and obstacles. Practice and Policy Guidelines Panel. Arch Fam Med 1997;6:149–54.
[3] Eisenberg DM, Kessler RC, Foster C, et al. Unconventional medicine in the United States: prevalence, costs, and patterns of use. N Engl J Med 1993;328:246–52.
[4] Krippner S. A cross cultural comparison of four healing models. Alternative therapies. Health and Medicine 1995;1:21–9.
[5] Mischoulon D. Nutraceuticals in psychiatry, part 1: social, technical, economic, and political perspectives. Contemporary Psychiatry 2004;2(11):1–6.
[6] Mischoulon D. Nutraceuticals in psychiatry, part 2: review of six popular psychotropics. Contemporary Psychiatry 2004;3(1):1–8.
[7] National Institutes of Health Office of Alternative Medicine. Alternative medicine: expanding medical horizons. Rockville (MD): National Institutes of Health Office of Alternative Medicine; 1992.
[8] Muller-Kuhrt L, Boesel R. Analysis of hypericins in hypericum extract. Nervenheilkunde 1993;12:359–61.
[9] Staffeldt B, Kerb R, Brockmoller J, et al. Pharmacokinetics of hypericin and pseudohypericin after oral intake of the Hypericum perforatum extract LI 160 in healthy volunteers. Nervenheilkunde 1993;12:331–8.
[10] Wagner H, Bladt S. Pharmaceutical quality of hypericum extracts. Nervenheilkunde 1993;12:362–6.
[11] Müller W, Rossol R. Effects of hypericum extract on the expression of serotonin receptors. Nervenheilkunde 1993;12:357–8.
[12] Thiele B, Ploch M, Brink I. Modulation of cytokine expression by hypericum extract. Nevenheilkunde 1993;12:353–6.
[13] Teufel-Mayer R, Gleitz J. Effects of long-term administration of hypericum extracts on the affinity and density of the central serotonergic 5-HT1 A and 5-HT2 A receptors. Pharmacopsychiatry 1997;30(Suppl 2):113–6.
[14] Nierenberg AA, Mischoulon D, DeCecco L. St. John's Wort: a critique of antidepressant efficacy and possible mechanisms of action. In: Mischoulon D, Rosenbaum J, editors. Natural medications for psychiatric disorders: considering the alternatives. Philadelphia: Lippincott Williams & Wilkins; 2002. p. 3–12.
[15] Laakmann G, Schule C, Baghai T, et al. St. John's Wort in mild to moderate depression: the relevance of hyperforin for the clinical efficacy. Pharmacopsychiatry 1998;31(Suppl 1):54–9.

[16] Orth HC, Rentel C, Schmidt PC. Isolation, purity analysis and stability of hyperforin as a standard material from Hypericum perforatum L. J Pharm Pharmacol 1999;51(2):193–200.

[17] Bladt S, Wagner H. MAO inhibition by fractions and constituents of hypericum extract. Nervenheilkunde 1993;12:349–52.

[18] Linde K, Mulrow CD, Berner M, et al. St John's wort for depression. Cochrane Database Syst Rev 2005;(2):CD000448.

[19] Vorbach EU, Hubner WD, Arnoldt KH. Effectiveness and tolerance of the hypericum extract LI 160 in comparison with imipramine. Randomized double blind study with 135 outpatients. Nevernheilkunde 1993;12:290–6. Also in J Geriatr Psychiatry Neurol 1994 Oct;7 Suppl 1:S19–23.

[20] Harrer G, Hubner WD, Podzuweit H. Effectiveness and tolerance of the hypericum preparation LI 160 compared to maprotiline. Multicentre double-blind study with 102 outpatients. Nervenheilkunde 1993;12:297–301.

[21] Martinez B, Kasper S, Ruhrmann B, et al. Hypericum in the treatment of seasonal affective disorders. Nervenheilkunde 1993;12:302–7.

[22] Wheatley D. LI 160, an extract of St. John's wort, versus amitriptyline in mildly to moderately depressed outpatients–a controlled 6-week clinical trial. Pharmacopsychiatry 1997; 30(Suppl 2):77–80.

[23] Nierenberg AA. St. John's Wort: a putative over-the-counter herbal antidepressant. Journal of Depressive Disorders, Index & Reviews 1998;III:16–7.

[24] Linde K, Ramirez G, Mulrow CD, et al. St. John's wort for depression–an overview and meta-analysis of randomized clinical trials. Br Med J 1996;313:253–8.

[25] Volz HP. Controlled clinical trials of hypericum extracts in depressed patients—an overview. Pharmacopsychiatry 1997;30(Suppl 2):72–6.

[26] Lecrubier Y, Clerc G, Didi R, et al. Efficacy of St. John's wort extract WS 5570 in major depression: a double-blind, placebo-controlled trial. Am J Psychiatry 2002;159(8):1361–6.

[27] Shelton RC, Keller MB, Gelenberg A, et al. Effectiveness of St John's wort in major depression: a randomized controlled trial. JAMA 2001;285(15):1978–86.

[28] Brenner R, Azbel V, Madhusoodanan S, et al. Comparison of an extract of hypericum (LI 160) and sertraline in the treatment of depression: a double-blind, randomized pilot study. Clin Ther 2000;22(4):411–9.

[29] Gastpar M, Singer A, Zeller K. Efficacy and tolerability of hypericum extract STW3 in long-term treatment with a once-daily dosage in comparison with sertraline. Pharmacopsychiatry 2005;38(2):78–86.

[30] van Gurp G, Meterissian GB, Haiek LN, et al. St John's wort or sertraline? Randomized controlled trial in primary care. Can Fam Physician 2002;48:905–12.

[31] Schrader E. Equivalence of St John's wort extract (Ze 117) and fluoxetine: a randomized, controlled study in mild-moderate depression. Int Clin Psychopharmacol 2000;15(2):61–8.

[32] Behnke K, Jensen GS, Graubaum HJ, et al. Hypericum perforatum versus fluoxetine in the treatment of mild to moderate depression. Adv Ther 2002;19(1):43–52.

[33] Hypericum Depression Trial Study Group. Effect of Hypericum perforatum (St John's wort) in major depressive disorder: a randomized controlled trial. JAMA 2002;287:1807–14.

[34] Fava M, Alpert J, Nierenberg AA, et al. A double-blind, randomized trial of St. John's Wort, fluoxetine, and placebo in major depressive disorder. J Clin Psychopharmacol 2005;25(5): 441–7.

[35] Moreno RA, Teng CT, Almeida KM, et al. Hypericum perforatum versus fluoxetine in the treatment of mild to moderate depression: a randomized double-blind trial in a Brazilian sample. Rev Bras Psiquiatr 2006;28(1):29–32 [Epub 2006 Mar 24].

[36] Baede-van Dijk PA, van Galen E, Lekkerkerker JF. [Drug interactions of Hypericum perforatum (St. John's wort) are potentially hazardous]. Ned Tijdschr Geneeskd 2000;144(17): 811–2. (Article in Dutch).

[37] Miller LG. Herbal medicinals: selected clinical considerations focusing on known or potential drug-herb interactions. Arch Intern Med 1998;158:2200–11.

[38] Moore LB, Goodwin B, Jones SA, et al. St. John's wort induces hepatic drug metabolism through activation of the pregnane X receptor. Proc Natl Acad Sci U S A 2000;97(13): 7500–2.

[39] Miller JL. Interaction between indinavir and St. John's wort reported. Am J Health Syst Pharm 2000;57(7):625–6.

[40] Piscitelli SC, Burstein AH, Chaitt D, et al. Indinavir concentrations and St John's wort. Lancet 2000;355(9203):547–8.

[41] Hu Z, Yang X, Ho PC, et al. Herb-drug interactions: a literature review. Drugs 2005;65(9): 1239–82.

[42] Schulz V. Safety of St. John's Wort extract compared to synthetic antidepressants. Phytomedicine 2006;13(3):199–204 [Epub 2005 Nov 2].

[43] Woelk H, Burkhard G, Grunwald J. Evaluation of the benefits and risks of the hypericum extract LI 160 based on a drug monitoring study with 3250 patients. Nervenheilkunde 1993;12:308–13.

[44] Beattie PE, Dawe RS, Traynor NJ, et al. Can St John's wort (hypericin) ingestion enhance the erythemal response during high-dose ultraviolet A1 therapy? Br J Dermatol 2005;153(6): 1187–91.

[45] Brockmoller J, Reum T, Bauer S, et al. Hypericin and pseudohypericin: pharmacokinetics and effects on photosensitivity in humans. Pharmacopsychiatry 1997;30(Suppl 2): 94–101.

[46] Siegers CP, Biel S, Wilhelm KP. Phototoxicity caused by hypericum. Nervenheilkunde 1993;12:320–2.

[47] Stevinson C, Ernst E. Can St. John's wort trigger psychoses? Int J Clin Pharmacol Ther 2004;42(9):473–80.

[48] Spillmann M, Fava M. S-adenosyl-methionine (ademethionine) in psychiatric disorders. CNS Drugs 1996;6:416–25.

[49] Alpert JE, Mischoulon D, Nierenberg AA, et al. Nutrition and depression: focus on folate. Nutrition 2000;16:544–6.

[50] Coppen A, Bailey J. Enhancement of the antidepressant action of fluoxetine by folic acid: a randomised, placebo controlled trial. J Affect Disord 2000;60:121–30.

[51] Alpert JE, Mischoulon D, Rubenstein GEF, et al. Folinic acid (Leucovorin) as an adjunctive treatment for SSRI-refractory depression. Ann Clin Psychiatry 2002;14:33–8.

[52] Fava M, Borus JS, Alpert JE, et al. Folate, B12, and homocysteine in major depressive disorder. Am J Psychiatr 1997;154:426–8.

[53] Bottiglieri T, Godfrey P, Flynn T, et al. Cerebrospinal fluid s-adenosylmethionine in depression and dementia: effects of treatment with parenteral and oral s-adenosylmethionine. J Neurol Neurosurg Psychiatr 1990;53:1096–8.

[54] Bell KM, Potkin SG, Carreon D, et al. S-adenosylmethionine blood levels in major depression: changes with drug treatment. Acta Neurol Scand Suppl 1994;154:15–8.

[55] Bottiglieri T, Chary TK, Laundy M, et al. Transmethylation in depression. Ala J Med Sci 1988;25:296–301.

[56] Matthysse S, Baldessarini RJ. S-adenosylmethionine and catechol-O-methyl-transferase in schizophrenia. Am J Psychiatry 1972;128:1310–2.

[57] Tolbert LC. MAT kinetics in affective disorders and schizophrenia. An account. Ala J Med Sci 1988;25:291–6.

[58] Bressa GM. S-Adenosyl-l-Methionine (SAMe) as antidepressant: meta-analysis of clinical studies. Acta Neurol Scand 1994;154(Suppl):7–14.

[59] Papakostas GI, Alpert JE, Fava M. S-Adenosyl methionine in depression: a comprehensive review of the literature. Curr Psychiatry Rep 2003;5:460–6.

[60] Mischoulon D, Fava M. Role of S-adenosyl-L-methionine in the treatment of depression: a review of the evidence. Am J Clin Nutr 2002;76(5 Suppl):1158S–61S.

[61] Fava M, Giannelli A, Rapisarda V, et al. Rapidity of onset of the antidepressant effect of parenteral S-adenosyl-L-methionine. Psychiatry Res 1995;56:295–7.

[62] Alvarez E, Udina C, Guillamat R. Shortening of latency period in depressed patients treated with SAMe and other antidepressant drugs. Cell Biol Rev 1987;S1:103–10.

[63] Berlanga C, Ortega-Soto HA, Ontiveros M, et al. Efficacy of S-adenosyl-L-methionine in speeding the onset of action of imipramine. Psychiatry Res 1992;44:257–62.

[64] Alpert JE, Papakostas G, Mischoulon D, et al. S-adenosyl-L-methionine (SAMe) as an adjunct for resistant major depressive disorder: an open trial following partial or nonresponse to selective serotonin reuptake inhibitors or venlafaxine. J Clin Psychopharmacol 2004;24(6): 661–4.

[65] Carney MWP, Chary TNK, Bottiglieri T. Switch mechanism in affective illness and oral S-adenosylmethionine (SAM). Br J Psychiatry 1987;150:724–5.

[66] Carney MW, Martin R, Bottiglieri T, et al. Switch mechanism in affective illness and S-adenosylmethionine. Lancet 1983;1:820–1.

[67] Adams PB, Lawson S, Sanigorski A, et al. Arachidonic acid to eicosapentaenoic acid ration in blood correlates positively with clinical symptoms of depression. Lipids 1996;31: 157–61.

[68] Hibbeln JR, Salem N Jr. Dietary polyunsaturated fatty acids and depression: when cholesterol does not satisfy. Am J Clin Nutr 1995;62:1–9.

[69] Cross-National Collaborative Group. The changing rate of major depression: cross national comparisons. JAMA 1992;268:3098–105.

[70] Hibbeln JR. Fish consumption and major depression [letter]. Lancet 1998;351:1213.

[71] Hibbeln JR. Long-chain polyunsaturated fatty acids in depression and related conditions. In: Peet M, Glen I, Horrobin DF, editors. Phospholipid spectrum disorder in psychiatry. Carnforth (UK): Marius Press; 1999. p. 195–210.

[72] Stoll AL, Locke CA. Omega-3 fatty acids in mood disorders: a review of neurobiological and clinical actions. In: Mischoulon D, Rosenbaum J, editors. Natural medications in psychiatric disorders. Philadelphia: Lippincott Williams & Wilkins; 2002. p. 13–34.

[73] Hamazaki K, Itomura M, Huan M, et al. Effect of omega-3 fatty acid-containing phospholipids on blood catecholamine concentrations in healthy volunteers: a randomized, placebo-controlled, double-blind trial. Nutrition 2005;21(6):705–10.

[74] Murck H, Song C, Horrobin DF, et al. Ethyl-eicosapentaenoate and dexamethasone resistance in therapy-refractory depression. Int J Neuropsychopharmacol 2004;7(3):341–9.

[75] Peet M, Horrobin DF. A dose-ranging study of the effects of ethyl-eicosapentaenoate in patients with ongoing depression despite apparently adequate treatment with standard drugs. Arch Gen Psychiatry 2002;59(10):913–9.

[76] Su KP, Huang SY, Chiu CC, et al. Omega-3 fatty acids in major depressive disorder. A preliminary double-blind, placebo-controlled trial. Eur Neuropsychopharmacol 2003;13(4): 267–71.

[77] Nemets B, Stahl ZM, Belmaker RH. Addition of omega-3 fatty acid to maintenance medication treatment for recurrent unipolar depressive disorder. Am J Psychiatry 2002;159: 477–9.

[78] Frangou S, Lewis M, McCrone P. Efficacy of ethyl-eicosapentaenoic acid in bipolar depression: randomised double-blind placebo-controlled study. Br J Psychiatry 2006;188:46–50.

[79] Silvers KM, Woolley CC, Hamilton FC, et al. Randomized double-blind placebo-controlled trial of fish oil in the treatment of depression. Prostaglandins Leukot Essent Fatty Acids 2005;72:211–8.

[80] Marangell LB, Martinez JM, Zboyan HA, et al. A double-blind, placebo-controlled study of the omega-3 fatty acid docosahexaenoic acid in the treatment of major depression. Am J Psychiatry 2003;160(5):996–8.

[81] Freeman MP, Hibbeln JR, Wisner KL, et al. Randomized dose-ranging pilot trial of omega-3 fatty acids for postpartum depression. Acta Psychiatr Scand 2006;113(1):31–5.

[82] Marangell LB, Martinez JM, Zboyan HA, et al. Omega-3 fatty acids for the prevention of postpartum depression: negative data from a preliminary, open-label pilot study. Depress Anxiety 2004;19(1):20–3.

[83] Stoll AL, Severus EW, Freeman MP, et al. Omega3 fatty acids in bipolar disorder: a preliminary double-blind, placebo-controlled trial. Arch Gen Psychiatry 1999;56:407–12.

[84] Keck PE Jr, Mintz J, McElroy SL, et al. Double-blind, randomized, placebo-controlled trials of ethyl-eicosapentanoate in the treatment of bipolar depression and rapid cycling bipolar disorder. Biol Psychiatry 2006;60:1020–2.

[85] Parker G, Gibson NA, Brotchie H, et al. Omega-3 fatty acids and mood disorders. Am J Psychiatry 2006;163(6):969–78.

[86] Osher Y, Bersudsky Y, Belmaker RH. Omega-3 eicosapentaenoic acid in bipolar depression: report of a small open-label study. J Clin Psychiatry 2005;66(6):726–9.

[87] Zanarini MC, Frankenburg FR. Omega-3 fatty acid treatment of women with borderline personality disorder: a double-blind, placebo-controlled pilot study. Am J Psychiatry 2003; 160:167–9.

[88] Mellor JE, Laugharne JDE, Peet M. Omega-3 fatty acid supplementation in schizophrenic patients. Hum Psychopharmacol 1996;11:39–46.

[89] Vaddadi KS, Courtney T, Gilleard CJ, et al. A double-blind trial of essential fatty acid supplementation in patients with tardive dyskinesia. Psychiatry Res 1989;27:313–23.

[90] Emsley R, Myburgh C, Oosthuizen P, et al. Randomized, placebo-controlled study of ethyl-eicosapentaenoic acid as supplemental treatment in schizophrenia. Am J Psychiatry 2002;159:1596–8.

[91] Fenton WS, Dickerson F, Boronow J, et al. A placebo-controlled trial of omega-3 fatty acid (ethyl eicosapentaenoic acid) supplementation for residual symptoms and cognitive impairment in schizophrenia. Am J Psychiatry 2001;158:2071–4.

[92] Maidment ID. Are fish oils an effective therapy in mental illness—an analysis of the data. Acta Psychiatr Scand 2000;102:3–11.

[93] Fux M, Benjamin J, Nemets B. A placebo-controlled cross-over trial of adjunctive EPA in OCD. J Psychiatr Res 2004;38(3):323–5.

[94] Peet M, Brind J, Ramchand CN, et al. Two double-blind placebo-controlled pilot studies of eicosapentaenoic acid in the treatment of schizophrenia. Schizophr Res 2001;49(3): 243–51.

[95] Freeman MP, Hibbeln JR, Wisner KL, et al. Omega-3 fatty acids: evidence basis for treatment and future research in psychiatry. J Clin Psychiatr 2006;67:1954–67.

[96] Chiu C-C, Huang S-Y, Shen WW, et al. Omega-3 fatty acids for depression in pregnancy [letter]. Am J Psychiatry 2003;160:385.

[97] Eisenberg DM. Advising patients who seek alternative medical therapies. Ann Intern Med 1997;127(1):61–9.

[98] Mischoulon D, Rosenbaum JF. The use of natural medications in psychiatry: a commentary. Harv Rev Psychiatry 1999;6:279–83.

Psychiatr Clin N Am 30 (2007) 69–76

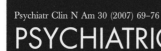

PSYCHIATRIC CLINICS
OF NORTH AMERICA

Comorbid Alcohol and Substance Abuse Dependence in Depression: Impact on the Outcome of Antidepressant Treatment

Michael J. Ostacher, MD, MPH[a,b,*]

[a]Department of Psychiatry, Harvard Medical School, Boston, MA, USA
[b]Department of Psychiatry, Massachusetts General Hospital, 50 Staniford Street, Suite 580, Boston, MA 02114, USA

M ajor depressive disorder often co-occurs with substance-use disorders, especially alcohol-use disorders [1–3], and the course of each of these problems seems be complicated by the other. Patients who have these comorbid conditions tend to be more severely depressed and impaired than those who have major depression alone; diagnosing and treating these patients is challenging [1,4]. A significant difficulty for clinicians is deciding whether treat a mood episode in a patient who has current substance use or a substance-use disorder and what is the optimal treatment.

It is not certain how these illnesses came to be viewed as separate, independent entities. This distinction may in large part result from the history of the treatment of substance abuse: in an era dominated by the psychoanalytically oriented treatment of mental illness, substance-use disorders often were not considered amenable to treatment. In that context, and with the rise of self-help programs such as Alcoholics Anonymous, addictions came to be treated in medical and community settings rather than by psychiatrists. Current evidence points to the co-occurrence of alcohol- and substance-use disorders as a common, expectable problem, with interactive effects between substance use and mood probably responsible for a more difficult course of illness, and to the possibility of shared genetic vulnerabilities [1,5,6,7]. In this context, however, little evidence is available to guide the clinician in using pharmacologic approaches in patients who have these comorbidities.

*Department of Psychiatry, Massachusetts General Hospital, 50 Staniford Street, Suite 580, Boston, MA 02114. E-mail address: mostacher@partners.org

0193-953X/07/$ – see front matter
doi:10.1016/j.psc.2006.12.009

PREVALENCE OF DEPRESSIVE AND SUBSTANCE-USE DISORDERS

Substance use can cause depressive and other psychiatric symptoms. This phenomenon has led to the development of diagnoses such as "Substance (or Alcohol) Induced Mood Disorder," which suggest that the psychiatric symptoms are caused the substance and not by any underlying psychiatric illness. Recent data, however, bring into question the clinical utility of such a concept, suggesting that patients who have substance-induced mood disorders (in which the symptoms of major depression occur during the course of substance use) are just as likely in prospective follow-up to have mood episodes independent of any substance use as are patients who have independent mood disorders and who have substance-use disorders [8]. For both groups, recurrence of depression is common and is most likely to occur independent of substance abuse. Even those patients whose history of alcohol use is in the past are perhaps four times as likely as those in the general population to have an episode of major depression [9,10]. These data underscore the importance of understanding whether treatment of depression in these patients will have a beneficial outcome.

It has been suggested that about 60% of mood disorders in individuals who have substance- or alcohol-use disorders are substance-induced (ie, occur exclusively during drug or alcohol use) rather than independent mood disorders [2,3,11,12], but more recent epidemiologic studies suggest instead that most mood disorders are independent of substance use. Grant and colleagues [1] have completed an ambitious study of the epidemiology of substance use and mental disorders, using methodology that more accurately diagnoses abuse and dependence syndromes and that carefully differentiates between independent and substance-induced mood disorders in adults. The National Institute on Alcohol Abuse and Alcoholism's National Epidemiologic Survey on Alcohol and Related Conditions (NESARC) is the largest comorbidity study completed to date, including data from 43,093 participants. The investigators found that an extraordinary proportion of adults who have substance or alcohol dependence and abuse have had independent mood episodes in the prior year and in their lifetimes. In the United States population, approximately 9% (19.2 million persons) had an independent mood disorder in the prior year, and about 9% (19.4 million) had a substance-use disorder. About 20% of individuals who have a current substance-use disorder had at least one current independent mood disorder, and 20% of individuals who had an independent mood disorder had at least one current substance-use disorder. Furthermore, few people had only substance-induced mood disorders.

In treatment-seeking populations, probably because of the increased severity and impairment found in patients who have both disorders, the proportions of depressed patients who have alcohol and drug misuse is higher than in the general population. In treatment-seeking populations in the NESARC sample, 20% of people who had independent mood disorders had a current substance-use disorder, but the proportions of people who had substance-use disorders seeking treatment who had an independent mood disorder were striking: more than 40% of people who had an alcohol-use disorder and 60% of those who had a substance-use disorder met criteria for an independent mood episode [1].

A recent systematic review of studies examining the association between alcohol problems and major depression found a median prevalence of current alcohol problems of 16% and a lifetime median prevalence of 30% in the population with major depression. In general population studies, alcohol abuse is about three times as common as alcohol dependence, although two thirds of respondents who have major depressive disorder and who have an alcohol-use disorder have alcohol dependence [1,13], suggesting a strong association between more severe alcohol problems and depression. In the Sequential Treatment Alternatives to Relieve Depression (STAR*D) trial, for instance, 29.4% of subjects who had major depressive disorder met criteria for concurrent substance-use disorder [7].

COURSE OF ILLNESS OF COMORBID DEPRESSION AND SUBSTANCE-USE DISORDERS

Comorbidity is associated with increased frequency of episodes, severity of depressive symptoms, lower functioning, and increased suicidality [7]. Depression, treated or not, strongly predicts relapse to drinking in alcohol-dependent persons [14], and the same seems to be true for substance-use disorders [10]. As mentioned previously, even a remote history of alcohol-use disorders is associated with depressive episodes [9].

In one study, depressed persons who had a history of alcohol dependence were more likely to report a history of childhood abuse, cigarette smoking, and suicide attempts than depressed persons who did not have a history of substance abuse, and these differences seems to be related to more aggressive traits on rating scales in the patients who had a history of alcohol-use disorder [15]. This finding raises the important question of whether the problems associated with illness course in patients who have this comorbidity are caused by factors other than substance use itself. In the STAR*D trial, chronicity of depression, defined as a baseline episode of depression lasting longer than 24 months, was not associated with alcohol or substance use [16]. Instead, generalized anxiety disorder, prior suicide attempts, fewer prior episodes, ill health, poverty, and being a member of a minority group were associated with persistent symptoms.

TREATMENT RESPONSE

Several methodologic issues complicate the interpretation of the data from studies of the treatment of mood disorders in patients who have current substance-use disorders. First, in an effort to increase the internal validity of the trials, virtually all large, placebo-controlled trials of antidepressants for major depression exclude persons who have current substance-use disorders (whether dependence or abuse). The vast data for modern and older antidepressants are of no help in predicting outcome for patients who have depression and substance-use disorder. Second, the studies of depression in subjects who have alcohol- and substance-use disorders generally include subjects who have dependence—not abuse—syndromes and may not represent the population of patients who have co-occurring substance-use and mood disorders who seek treatment in primary care and general psychiatric treatment settings. This limitation, however, is not uniform across studies. Outcomes from these studies may provide little direct evidence for the treatment of patients who have substance-abuse rather than substance-dependence diagnoses. Third, there is not a uniform definition of depression across studies; some studies include only subjects who have a research diagnosis of major depressive disorder with a minimum score on a depression rating scale; others include subjects who have major depressive disorder, dysthymia, and depression not otherwise specified (NOS). This heterogeneity makes comparisons between trials difficult and limits the generalizability of the results. Finally, some studies include subjects who are not abstinent from drugs or alcohol at entry into the trial; others include only subjects who have been detoxified in inpatient settings and are abstinent at the start of treatment.

There are a myriad of published reports of the treatment of depression in patients who have substance-use disorders, ranging from case reports to moderately large, randomized, placebo-controlled trials. Unfortunately, there are few well-designed, adequately powered trials to guide clinicians and patients in the treatment of depression comorbid with substance or alcohol problems. A systematic review and meta-analysis of antidepressant treatment of depressed patients who have alcohol or substance misuse published by Nunes and Levin [17] is the best attempt to date to examine and interpret the current data. This review found that antidepressant treatment had an overall modest effect on depressive symptoms in patients who had co-occurring unipolar depressive disorders (major depressive disorder, dysthymia, and depression NOS) and drug- and alcohol-use disorder and a small effect in decreasing drug or alcohol use in these subjects. They found that the likelihood of finding an antidepressant effect was higher in studies with low placebo response (consistent with findings in antidepressant trials in subjects without substance abuse) and concluded that antidepressants can be useful in these patients if used in adequate doses, for an adequate length of time (at least 6 weeks), and in patients whose diagnosis is well established by a thorough history and a structured diagnostic interview. The overall effect size they found was 0.38 (95% confidence interval [CI], 0.18–0.58), which compares favorably with the effect size, 0.43, found in a meta-analysis of antidepressant trials in unipolar depression.

Antidepressant efficacy was greater in patients who had alcohol-use disorder than in those who had substance-use disorder, but the effect in subjects who had substance-use disorder was still significant. Strikingly, the extent of placebo response was the variable that accounted for most of the difference between positive and negative trials. In studies with placebo response rates greater than 25%, there was almost no difference between drug and placebo, but in studies with placebo response rates lower than 25%, the effect size was large

(0.68; 95% CI, 0.49–0.88). As expected, the inclusion of psychosocial treatment in a study diminished the drug–placebo difference.

The largest study of major depression with alcohol dependence, which was published after the meta-analysis by Nunes and Levin [17], compared sertraline with placebo in 328 subjects. This study found no additional benefit of the drug compared with placebo [18]. In both groups response rates were greater than 50%. The study was limited primarily by the overall low severity of depression of the subjects, with an mean baseline score on the 17-item Hamilton Depression Scale of 17.2. Although this study was intended to address many of the methodologic concerns that limited the usefulness of earlier studies, ultimately it, too, was hampered by an additional methodologic flaw: subjects were included if they met criteria for a major depressive episode after only 4 days of abstinence. It thus included a large number of subjects whose depressive symptoms might have resolved spontaneously during a longer period of abstinence. The overall low severity of symptoms coupled with the high placebo response rate led to a failed trial. The authors did attempt to examine subgroups of subjects who had high depression scale scores and found no significant benefit for sertraline, but the number of subjects in this group was too small for the finding to be definitive.

Although the available evidence from clinical trials of antidepressant treatments of comorbid depression and substance-use disorders is limited, efforts to increase antidepressant prescribing and adherence do seem to have a positive benefit on depression outcomes in patients who have comorbid substance and alcohol use, supporting the conclusion of Nunes and coworkers [17], that antidepressants are helpful in the treatment of these patients [17,19]. Watkins and colleagues [19] published data from a large, randomized trial comparing a quality-improvement intervention in a primary care setting (n = 1356) and compared outcomes of depression treatment for patients with and without comorbid substance misuse. Although, as expected, the group with substance misuse and depression had more severe symptoms both at baseline and follow-up; there was not a differential effect based on comorbidity. In each cohort, the patients who received the quality improvement intervention (supervision, review of cases and education for clinic staff, and psychoeducation for patients) had better outcomes than the patients who received usual care. For those who had comorbid substance misuse, depression outcomes were improved at 12 months, and antidepressant use was increased at 6 months compared with the usual-care group; in the group without substance misuse, depression outcomes were improved at 6 months. This quality-improvement study found that the interventions that improve outcomes for depression—primarily increased prescribing and patient counseling to improve adherence—do so whether or not the depression is complicated by substance or alcohol use.

Small continuation studies support continued use of antidepressants in this group, although the data are not definitive. Cornelius and colleagues [20] followed 31 subjects naturalistically after a placebo-controlled trial comparing fluoxetine with placebo in comorbid alcohol dependence and depression, finding that the fluoxetine group had lower depression and drinking severity at 1-year follow-up.

Participants STAR*D trial were not excluded from participation because of substance-use disorders. These patients tended to be a more ill group, with more episodes and earlier age of onset of mood disorder. Outcome data from this subset of study participants have not been published yet but may provide real-world evidence of effectiveness for the treatment of co-occurring mood and substance-use disorders.

SUMMARY

Substance and alcohol problems frequently co-occur with major depressive disorder, and these comorbid conditions are associated with greater severity of illness and rate of recurrence for both disorders. Perhaps because of value judgments about people's behavior with regards to drug and alcohol use (unlike, say, attitudes about anxiety disorders, which also are associated with poor outcome in depression), compounded by the mistaken impression that depression in most patients who have substance- and alcohol-use disorders is caused by the direct effects of substances, the discomfort of many clinicians when treating patients who use substances and alcohol has interfered with access to care. Although there are few definitive studies to guide clinician practice for the complicated clinical picture of patients presenting for treatment of depression comorbid with substance and alcohol misuse, abuse, and dependence, several treatment recommendations can be made based on the existing literature:

1. All patients who have depressive disorders should be screened carefully for the extent of their drug and alcohol use. Because of the high prevalence of the comorbidity of alcohol- and substance-use disorders in patients who have depression, all patients presenting with depressive symptoms should be questioned about their use of drugs and alcohol. Comorbidity is associated with more disability, depression severity, and history of suicide attempts, and interventions for this group should be more, rather than less, intensive.
2. Depression frequently is recurrent in patients who have comorbid substance use, and it is not clear that antidepressant treatment should be withheld from patients whose episodes of depression occur during periods of drug or alcohol use, because recurrence of independent depressive episodes is common. In patients who have a history of substance- and alcohol-use disorders, the course of illness does not seem to be significantly different whether an episode of depression is associated with drug or alcohol use or is independent of it; independent and substance-induced mood episodes are both most likely to recur independent of drug or alcohol use.
3. Treatment with antidepressant medication in these patients is associated with decreased depressive symptoms (for alcohol more than for other substances) and decreased substance use, although large trials of antidepressants for alcohol-dependent subjects who have depressive disorders have been hampered by high placebo response rates. In spite of the methodologic and practical barriers to conducting research specific to comorbid populations, there is a clear pattern

of benefit in favor of antidepressant drug treatment for patients who have co-occurring major depression and substance-use disorders. Selective serotonin reuptake inhibitors, mirtazapine, venlafaxine, nefazedone, and tricyclic antidepressants seem to be safe when used in depressed patients who have current drug- and alcohol-use disorders [17,20–23]. There is no evidence that current drug or alcohol use affects the safety of antidepressants in adults, and safety concerns about drug interactions may be a minimal concern.

4. Psychosocial treatment interventions to enhance medication use improve outcomes for patients who have comorbid conditions; the benefit of combined treatment is similarly large with major depression with or without substance abuse. To a great degree, medication adherence is associated with outcome for depression, and antidepressant adherence in the treatment of depression is associated with good outcome as much in patients who have substance use-disorders as in those who do not. Lack of adherence is not inevitable in the treatment of this comorbidity.

Patients who have drug- and alcohol-use disorder should be counseled about their use and should be referred for substance-abuse treatment if they are dependent or are unable to curtail their use during treatment. Interventions specific to substance use—as simple as education regarding the relationship between use and symptoms—should be recommended for these patients.

References

[1] Grant BF, Stinson FS, Dawson DA, et al. Prevalence and co-occurrence of substance use disorders and independent mood and anxiety disorders: results from the National Epidemiologic Survey on Alcohol and Related Conditions (NESARC). Arch Gen Psychiatry 2004;61:807–16.

[2] Kessler RC, Berglund P, Demler O, et al. National Comorbidity Survey Replication. The epidemiology of major depressive disorder: results from the National Comorbidity Survey Replication (NCS-R). JAMA 2003;289:3095–105.

[3] Kessler RC, Walters EE. The National Comorbidity Survey. In: Tsaung MT, Tohen M, editors. Textbook in psychiatric epidemiology. 2nd edition. New York: John Wiley & Sons Inc; 2002. p. 343–62.

[4] Sanderson K, Andrews G. Prevalence and severity of mental health disability and relationship to diagnosis. Psychiatr Serv 2002;53:80–6.

[5] Nurnberger JI Jr, Foroud T, Flury L, et al. Evidence for a locus on chromosome 1 that influences vulnerability to alcoholism and affective disorder. Am J Psychiatry 2001;158:718–24.

[6] Wang JC, Hinrichs AL, Stock H, et al. Evidence of common and specific genetic effects: association of the muscarinic acetylcholine receptor M2 (CHRM2) gene with alcohol dependence and major depressive syndrome. Hum Mol Genet 2004;13:1903–11.

[7] Davis LL, Rush JA, Wisniewski SR, et al. Substance use disorder comorbidity in major depressive disorder: an exploratory analysis of the Sequenced Treatment Alternatives to Relieve Depression cohort. Compr Psychiatry 2005;46:81–9.

[8] Nunes EV, Liu X, Samet S, et al. Independent versus substance-induced major depressive disorder in substance-dependent patients: observational study of course during follow-up. J Clin Psychiatry 2006;67:1561–7.

[9] Hasin DS, Grant BF. Major depression in 6,050 former drinkers. Arch Gen Psychiatry 2002;59:794–800.

[10] Hasin D, Liu X, Nunes E, et al. Effects of major depression on remission and relapse of substance dependence. Arch Gen Psychiatry 2002;59:375–80.

[11] Regier DA, Farmer ME, Rae DS, et al. Comorbidity of mental disorders with alcohol and other drug abuse: results from the Epidemiologic Catchment Area (ECA) Study. JAMA 1990;264:2511–8.

[12] Schuckit MA, Tipp JE, Bergman M, et al. Comparison of induced and independent major depressive disorder in 2,945 alcoholics. Am J Psychiatry 1997;154:948–57.

[13] Conway KP, Compton W, Stinson FS, Grant BF. Lifetime comorbidity of DSM-IV mood and anxiety disorders and specific drug use disorders: results from the National Epidemiologic Survey on Alcohol and Related Conditions. J Clin Psychiatry Feb 2006;67(2):247–57.

[14] Greenfield S, Weiss R, Nuenz L, et al. The effect of depression on return to drinking: a prospective study. Arch Gen Psychiatry 1998;55:269–265.

[15] Sher L, Oquendo MA, Galfalvy HC, et al. The relationship of aggression to suicidal behavior in depressed patients with a history of alcoholism. Addict Behav 2005;30:1144–53.

[16] Gilmer WS, Trivedi MH, Rush AJ, et al. Factors associated with chronic depressive episodes: a preliminary report from the STAR-D project. Acta Psychiatr Scand 2005;112:425–33.

[17] Nunes EV, Levin FR. Treatment of depression in patients with alcohol or other drug dependence: a meta-analysis. JAMA 2004;291:1887–96.

[18] Kranzler HR. Evidence-based treatments for alcohol dependence: new results and new questions. JAMA 2006;295:2075–6.

[19] Watkins KE, Paddock SM, Zhang L, et al. Improving care for depression in patients with comorbid substance misuse. Am J Psychiatry 2006;163:125–32.

[20] Cornelius JR, Salloum IM, Haskett RF, et al. Fluoxetine versus placebo in depressed alcoholics: a 1-year follow-up study. Addict Behav 2000;25:307–10.

[21] Mason BJ, Kocsis JH, Ritvo EC, et al. A double-blind, placebo-controlled trial of desipramine for primary alcohol dependence stratified on presence or absence of major depression. JAMA 1996;275:761–7.

[22] McGrath PJ, Nunes EV, Stewart JW, et al. Imipramine treatment of alcoholics with primary depression: a placebo-controlled clinical trial. Arch Gen Psychiatry 1996;53:232–40.

[23] Nunes EV, Quitkin FM, Donovan SJ, et al. Imipramine treatment of opiate-dependent patients with depressive disorders: a placebo-controlled trial. Arch Gen Psychiatry 1998;55:153–60.

Treating Depression in the Medically Ill

Dan V. Iosifescu, MD, MSc[a,b,*]

[a]Depression Clinical and Research Program, Massachusetts General Hospital, 50 Staniford Street, Suite 401, Boston, MA 02114, USA
[b]Harvard Medical School, Boston, MA, USA

A large body of evidence demonstrates the coexistence of depressive disorders and several medical illnesses. The comorbidity of depression and medical illness is important as it relates to the understanding of etiologic factors for each disease [1]. Moreover, there is a bidirectional relationship between depression and medical illnesses, each having a negative impact on prognosis and treatment of the other condition.

The comorbidity of depression and medical illness is not a new concept. As early as 1929 Gillespie [2] made a distinction between endogenous depressive disorders (such as depression associated with medical illness) and affective psychogenic disorders, providing specific criteria for distinguishing the two categories. Shortly thereafter, however, Lewis [3] found that these criteria failed to differentiate distinct disorders adequately and argued that depression is a continuum. In the 1970s, depression associated with medical illness was considered "secondary" or "reactive" (ie, a psychologic consequence of having an illness) and to have a less severe clinical course [4]. Several investigators, however, found very few and inconsistent differences in the clinical presentation of primary and secondary depression [5–7]. Currently, depression with comorbid medical illness is not considered a different diagnostic entity but a part of the continuum of symptoms of depressive disorders.

A significant number of studies, however, have focused on the impact of depression on the outcome of medical illness. In this context, the presence of depression was predictive of poor outcomes of the medical illness and of increased mortality. Such results were reported in depression associated with

Dr. Iosifescu has received research grant support from Aspect Medical Systems, Forest Laboratories, Janssen Pharmaceutica, NARSAD, and NIMH; he has been a consultant for Aspect Medical Systems, Forest Laboratories Inc., Gerson Lehrman Group, GlaxoSmithKline, and Pfizer Inc., and he has been a speaker for Eli Lilly & Company, Cephalon, Forest Laboratories Inc., Janssen Pharmaceutica, Organon Inc., and Pfizer Inc.

This work was supported by an NIMH K-23 Career Development Award (K23MH067111).

*Massachusetts General Hospital, 50 Staniford Street, Suite 401, Boston, MA 02114.
E-mail address: diosifescu@partners.org

0193-953X/07/$ – see front matter
doi:10.1016/j.psc.2006.12.008

cardiovascular disease [8–10], stroke [11,12], diabetes [13], and cancer [14]. Similar increases in mortality were reported in studies of depression associated with the overall burden of comorbid medical illness [15,16].

An equally important question pertains to the longitudinal course of depression in persons who have comorbid medical illness. To answer this question, the article reviews randomized, controlled studies of antidepressant treatment in patients who had major depressive disorder (MDD) and several medical comorbidities (myocardial infarction [MI], stroke, diabetes, cancer, and rheumatoid arthritis). It also reviews a series of studies comparing the outcome of antidepressant treatment in patients who have MDD with and without comorbid medical illness.

STUDIES ON THE PREVALENCE OF MAJOR DEPRESSIVE DISORDER IN MEDICALLY ILL SUBJECTS

A large number of studies have reported increased rates of MDD in subjects diagnosed with specific medical illnesses. Depression occurs in as many as 27% of patients after MI, and it impacts their recovery negatively [17]. Of patients hospitalized for acute MI, 18% were diagnosed with major depression, and 45% were diagnosed with major or minor depression [18,19]. In several studies, 25% to 32% of patients were diagnosed with MDD in the first year after MI [20,21]. The prevalence of MDD was 18% in patients who had coronary artery disease documented by coronary angiography [22] and 17% in patients during their first year after heart transplantation [23]. The prevalence of MDD also was increased in patients who had chronic heart failure [24,25]. Moreover, high rates of depression have been reported in association with the total burden of vascular risk factors [26] and in relation to individual vascular risk factors such as hypertension [27,28] and smoking [29,30]. Conversely, Wulsin and Singal [31], based on a meta-analysis of 11 large studies, estimated that depression increases the risk of coronary disease by 1.64-fold (95% confidence interval [CI], 1.41–1.90). The risk of cardiac death is increased by approximately fourfold in patients who have depression 6 months after an MI compared with nondepressed post-MI patients [8]; the post-MI mortality risk in depressed patients remains increased by 3.5-fold at 5 years after the MI [32].

In the immediate aftermath of a cerebrovascular accident (3–6 months after stroke), 20% to 30% of patients met criteria for MDD [33–35]. The prevalence of MDD remained 38% after 1 year [21] and 29% at 3 years after the stroke [34]. More recent pooled data from large studies conducted around the world reveal prevalence rates for major depression of 19.3% to 23.3% in post-stroke depression [36]. In patients who had suffered a stroke, depression at 1 month was associated with higher mortality at 12 months (odds ratio [OR] 3.1; 95% CI, 1.1–8.8) and at 24 months (OR 2.2; 95% CI, 1.0–4.8) [37]. In a large recent epidemiologic study Brown and co-workers [38] found an adjusted hazard ratio of 1.73 (95% CI, 1.20–2.66) for developing depression in subjects within 2 years after treatment for stroke. Moreover, in the large North East Melbourne Stroke Incidence Study, depression and anxiety were significant determinants of persistent handicap after a stroke [39].

Several studies have supported the hypothesis that depression contributes to hypertension [28,40,41]. Among 452 psychiatric outpatients, the prevalence of MDD was increased threefold in patients who had hypertension [27]. Bosworth and coworkers [28] reported the odds ratio for depressed patients being hypertensive was 2.13, compared with nondepressed patients.

Depression also may be associated similarly with ulcers [42]. Levenstein and collaborators [43] examined 4595 ulcer-free subjects and found a significant relationship between depression and later ulcer development.

Depression is common in patients who have diabetes. In a meta-analysis of 20 studies, Gavard and colleagues [44] reported that depression was three to four times more prevalent in patients who had diabetes than in the general population. In a meta-analysis of 42 studies [45], the odds of depression in the diabetes group were twice that of the nondiabetes group. The mean prevalence of depression in these studies was 14% (range, 9%–27%). Alternatively, a history of depression is associated with an increased risk of diabetes [46]. Moreover, the presence of depression has been associated with more diabetes-related complications [13] and with higher glycosylated hemoglobin levels [47].

A high prevalence of depression also has been described in patients who have cancer [14,48]. Depression may also be a consequence of antineoplastic therapies [49]. In a sample of 5000 elderly subjects, the presence of chronic depression was associated with an increased risk of cancer (hazard ratio, 1.88; 95% CI, 1.13–3.14) [50]. The presence of depression was associated with shortened survival times in patients who had cancer [14,49].

Increased prevalence of MDD has been reported in multiple studies of person who have multiple comorbid medical illnesses [51,52]. In a study of 2554 persons [53] the 6-month prevalence of depression increased from 6% to 9% when comorbid medical illness was present, and the lifetime prevalence increased from 9% to 13%. In a sample of 17,626 Canadians [54], several chronic medical conditions (asthma, chronic obstructive pulmonary disease [COPD], gastrointestinal ulcers, cancer, migraine, back pain) as well as the total burden of medical disease were associated with an elevated prevalence of major depression. Similarly, in a study of 2481 post-MI patients, the rates of major and minor depression were significantly higher in patients who had greater levels of medical comorbidity [55]. The association of depression and general medical comorbidity is significant because it defines a patient population with increased functional disability. In a survey of 130,880 Canadians, the presence of comorbid MDD was associated with increased functional disability and work absence compared with the presence of a chronic physical illness without comorbid MDD [56]. This impact of MDD was seen across each of the six chronic physical illnesses examined (heart disease, diabetes, arthritis, asthma, back problems, and COPD).

RANDOMIZED, CONTROLLED STUDIES OF ANTIDEPRESSANT TREATMENT IN MAJOR DEPRESSIVE DISORDER COMORBID WITH SPECIFIC MEDICAL ILLNESSES

Although antidepressant treatments and psychotherapies are effective in depressed medically ill patients, the efficacy of such treatments is lower in this population than in depressed individuals who are not medically ill. This point is illustrated by a review of a series of randomized studies in patients who had MDD and various medical comorbidities: MI, stroke, diabetes, cancer, and rheumatoid arthritis.

The Montreal Heart Attack Readjustment Trial [57] assigned 1376 post-MI patients randomly to an intervention program with repeated monitoring or to treatment as usual; no additional improvement in mortality was detected. The intervention had little effect on depression and anxiety scores compared with treatment as usual. Three controlled, randomized trials of antidepressants in patients after MI have been published in the last decade [58–60]. Two of these trials were placebo controlled [59,60]; one trial used an active comparator without placebo [58]. Both placebo-controlled trials failed to demonstrate an advantage of the antidepressant over placebo on the primary outcome measure. Secondary outcome measures in the Sertraline Antidepressant Heart Attack Randomized Trial [60] did show an advantage of sertraline over placebo in clinician global impression and in the subgroup of patients who had recurrent depression. Nelson and coworkers [58] reported significant improvement of depression with both paroxetine and nortriptyline, without any significant difference between the two. The Enhancing Recovery In Coronary Heart Disease [61] study randomly assigned 2481 post-MI subjects to cognitive behavioral therapy (CBT) versus treatment as usual. CBT produced modest but statistically significant improvements in depression and social support scores at 6 months after randomization. CBT did not increase survival, however. Of interest, patients in this study who received sertraline (not randomized) had a significantly lower risk of death or nonfatal MI (adjusted hazard ratio, 0.63; 95% CI, 0.46–0.87) [62].

Several randomized, placebo-controlled studies in the treatment of post-stroke depression have been published in the last 15 years [63–67]. One study [65] reported that fluoxetine was superior to placebo; in three other studies [64,66,67] fluoxetine did not separate from placebo. In one study each, nortriptyline [64] and citalopram [63] were superior to placebo for the treatment of MDD in poststroke patients. Other researchers attempted to use antidepressants to prevent poststroke depression [68,69]. One study [68] suggested nortriptyline and fluoxetine were equally efficacious and superior to placebo in preventing poststroke depression, but the nortriptyline-treated group had a higher rate of depressive relapse after treatment discontinuation. Sertraline, however, was reported not superior to placebo in preventing depression at the 6-month follow-up [69].

In a review of antidepressant studies for patients who had MDD and diabetes, Goodnick [70] observed that treatment with selective serotonin reuptake inhibitors improves depression and is associated with improved diabetes outcomes. Both nortriptyline [71] and fluoxetine [72] have been found superior to placebo for the treatment of depression in diabetes patients. Of note, Lustman and coworkers [72] detected an advantage for fluoxetine improving glycemic control for diabetes patients, whereas in their previous study nortriptyline worsened glycemic control [71]. CBT also is more effective that treatment as usual in treating depression in patients who have diabetes [73]; at 6 months follow-up mean glycosylated hemoglobin levels were significantly better in the CBT group than in the control group. More recently, the Pathways Study [74] randomly assigned 329 patients to either standard care or collaborative care (including antidepressant treatment or problem-solving therapy). Depression scores improved more in the collaborative-care intervention than in standard care, but this improvement did not translate to improved glycemic control in those subjects.

Williams and Dale [75] extensively reviewed published studies of pharmacologic and/or psychotherapy interventions in depressed patients who had cancer, concluding that antidepressants seem to be effective in reducing depression/depressive symptoms in these patients. In placebo-controlled trials mianserin [76], fluoxetine [77], and paroxetine [78,79] were all superior to placebo in the treatment of MDD in patients who had cancer. No significant difference was detected between fluoxetine and desipramine [80] or between amitriptyline and paroxetine [81], all treatments being equally useful for depression in patients who had cancer. The data on the efficacy of psychotherapeutic interventions in treating depression/depressive symptoms in patients who have cancer are more limited, but CBT seems to be effective in reducing depressive symptoms in this population [75].

In a randomized, controlled study the tricyclic antidepressant dothiepin was superior to placebo for the treatment of MDD with comorbid rheumatoid arthritis [82]. Both paroxetine and amitriptyline were found to be equally efficacious in this population, with no significant difference between them [83]. In a recent study, Parker and coworkers [84] reported that adding CBT did not improve the significant benefit of antidepressant medications.

STUDIES COMPARING TREATMENT OUTCOME IN MAJOR DEPRESSIVE DISORDER WITH AND WITHOUT COMORBID MEDICAL ILLNESS

Earlier studies of tricyclic antidepressants reported low rates of improvement of depressive symptoms in patients who had MDD and comorbid medical illness [85]. Most of these studies, however, used open designs with subtherapeutic doses of tricyclic antidepressants [85] because of the side effects and contraindications of tricyclic antidepressants in these severely ill populations [86].

Of eight more recent studies on the outcome of acute antidepressant treatment in patients who had MDD with and without medical illness [87–95], three studies were randomized and controlled [87–89,95], two studies had an open-label prospective design with one single antidepressant being used [93,94], and three other studies had naturalistic designs with a variety of antidepressants [87,91,92]. The diagnosis of depression was restricted to MDD in five studies [87–90,93–95], two studies focused on treatment-resistant MDD [93,95], and other two studies included MDD and other depressive disorders [91,92]. The ratings of the medical illness were done merely by noting the presence of medical illness [87,91], by the number of comorbid medical illnesses [88], by a severity rating (mild, moderate, severe) of comorbid medical illness [89,90], by organ systems affected by medical illness [92], or by using a rating scale for the severity of the comorbid illness [93–95]. Comparing the results is difficult because of the differences among studies. Five of the eight studies [87,89–92,94] reported lower treatment response in patients who had MDD and comorbid medical illness. Of the three studies [88,93,95] reporting no difference in treatment outcome in patients with and without medical comorbidity, two studies [93,95] included only patients who had treatment-resistant MDD and had small numbers (n = 92 and n = 101), thus having small power to detect a difference.

Fewer studies compared antidepressant treatment for prevention of MDD relapse in patients with and without comorbid medical illness [96,97]. In a group of 128 subjects who responded to antidepressant treatment, higher medical comorbidity (measured with the Cumulative Illness Rating Scale [CIRS]) was predictive of higher rates of relapse during continuation treatment with fluoxetine and with increases in self-reported symptoms of depression, anxiety, and anger [97]. In a smaller study (n = 58) no significant relationship was detected between medical comorbidity (CIRS score) and MDD relapse or recurrence during treatment with nortriptyline [96]. In an observational study of primary care patients beginning antidepressant treatment [98], patients who had medical illness (ischemic heart disease, diabetes, or COPD) showed significant improvement of depression over 6 months, but the rate of improvement was slower in patients who had heart disease.

More recently two large, randomized studies compared the effectiveness of collaborative treatments (including antidepressant management and/or psychotherapy, case management, and education) with standard care in the treatment of depressed medically ill individuals. Among the 324 elderly persons (age > 60 years) randomly assigned in the Prevention of Suicide in Primary Care Elderly: Collaborative Trial (PROSPECT) study [99] none of the comorbid medical conditions were associated with outcomes of depression treatment in the intervention group, but specific medical illnesses were associated with outcomes in the usual care group. In the Improving Mood-Promoting Access to Collaborative Treatment (IMPACT) study [100] among 1801 depressed older adults (age >60 years), those randomly assigned to the intervention had lower depression scores, but the number of chronic diseases did not affect the likelihood of response to the intervention.

In conclusion, most studies suggest that depressed medically ill individuals may be more treatment refractory, respond slower or less well to antidepressant treatment, and have higher rates of depressive relapse in the continuation phase. Other studies [99,100] suggest that more intensive collaborative treatments, including antidepressants, psychotherapy, education, and case management, can be effective in this treatment-refractory population.

PUTATIVE MECHANISMS OF THE INTERACTION BETWEEN DEPRESSION AND MEDICAL ILLNESS

There are several hypotheses regarding the mechanism by which medical illness can affect clinical response in MDD. Ciechanowski and collaborators [101] postulate that the relationship between medical illness and depressive symptoms may be mediated by factors such as self-care, nutrition, and adherence to treatment. Pharmacokinetic or pharmacodynamic properties of antidepressants may be changed in the context of comorbid medical illness or concurrent medications [102].

It has been postulated that the association between MDD and medical illness is mediated by stress and activation of the hypothalamic-pituitary-adrenal (HPA) axis [103]. Numerous studies have reported an excess of cortisol and nonsuppression in the dexamethasone suppression test (DST) in patients who have MDD. In a review of more than 150 studies, Arana and coworkers [104] reported that 43% of persons who had MDD (n = 4411) and 67% of persons who had psychotic depression (n = 150) were DST nonsuppressors. DST nonsuppression is correlated with worse clinical course in MDD (ie, a higher number of lifetime depressive episodes [105]) and with a higher risk of MDD relapse [106]. Despite their high level of cortisol at baseline, patients who have MDD continue to experience a degree of cortisol elevation after stress as high as that seen in normal controls, leading to a chronic state of hypercortisolemia [107]. High levels of cortisol and stress have been associated with neurotoxic changes in the hippocampus in animal models [108] and in subjects who have MDD [109,110]. Moreover, hypercortisolemia and excessive HPA-axis activation have been implicated in several chronic medical illnesses (eg, hypertension [111], gastrointestinal ulcers [112], and diabetes [113]) and with risk factors for vascular disease such as hypercholesterolemia [114]. Therefore, hypercholesterolemia and excessive HPA-axis activation can represent a common pathway for the interaction between depression and chronic medical illness, although this correlation has not yet been demonstrated.

Another hypothesis involves the role of cytokines, nonantibody proteins released by cells on contact with antigens [115]. Cytokines are increased in a variety of infectious and noninfectious illnesses that involve activation of the immune system. Noninfectious diseases associated with increased levels of cytokines include coronary artery disease [116,117], hypertension [118], other vascular atherosclerosis [119], COPD [120], diabetes [121], and arthritis and autoimmune diseases [122]. Further observations have shown that administration of cytokines such as interleukin 2, tumor necrosis factor, or interferon alfa may induce depressive symptoms [122,123]. The increased production of cytokines has further impact on cortisol production and on the HPA axis. Antidepressants also have been shown to reduce the immune response and to suppress cytokine production [122,124,125]. The association

between cytokine production and response rates in MDD is still unproven,
however.

SUMMARY

Depression frequently is comorbid with a variety of medical illnesses; individuals who have such comorbidities may have increased morbidity and lower
functional status.

Usual antidepressant treatments can be effective in depressed patients who
have comorbid medical illness. These patients, however, experience lower rates
of recovery and remission of depressive symptoms and higher rates of relapse
during follow-up than seen in patients who have MDD with no medical comorbidity. Comorbid medical illness therefore is a marker of treatment resistance
in MDD. Collaborative treatments combining antidepressants, psychotherapy,
education, and case management may be effective and could overcome the risk
of treatment resistance.

Two clinical strategies seem warranted in light of the studies presented here:
(1) an increased index of suspicion for depression in medically ill patients, and
(2) more intensive antidepressant treatment in depressed patients who have
medical comorbidity.

References

[1] Krishnan KR, Delong M, Kraemer H, et al. Comorbidity of depression with other medical
    diseases in the elderly. Biol Psychiatry 2002;52(6):559–88.
[2] Gillespie L. The clinical differentiation of types of depression. Guys Hosp rep 1929;79:
    231–3.
[3] Lewis A. Melancholia: a clinical survey of depressive states. J Ment Sci 1934;80:
    277–378.
[4] Klerman GL. Depression in the medically ill. Psychiatr Clin North Am 1981;4:301–17.
[5] Andreasen NC, Winokur G. Secondary depression: familial, clinical, and research per-
    spectives. Am J Psychiatry 1979;136(1):62–6.
[6] Akiskal HS, Rosenthal RH, Rosenthal TL, et al. Differentiation of primary affective illness
    from situational, symptomatic, and secondary depressions. Arch Gen Psychiatry 1979;
    36(6):635–43.
[7] Hirschfeld RM, Klerman GL, Andreasen NC, et al. Situational major depressive disorder.
    Arch Gen Psychiatry 1985;42(11):1109–14.
[8] Frasure-Smith N, Lesperance F, Talajic M. Depression following myocardial infarction.
    Impact on 6-month survival. JAMA 1993;270(15):1819–25.
[9] Frasure-Smith N, Lesperance F, Talajic M. Depression and 18-month prognosis after
    myocardial infarction. Circulation 1995;91(4):999–1005.
[10] Bush DE, Zigelstein RC, Tayback M, et al. Even minimal symptoms of depression
    increase mortality risk after acute myocardial infarction. Am J Cardiol 2001;88:
    337–41.
[11] Kauhanen M, Korpelainen JT, Hiltunen P, et al. Poststroke depression correlates with
    cognitive impairment and neurological deficits. Stroke 1999;30(9):1875–80.
[12] Jorge RE, Robinson RG, Arndt S, et al. Mortality and post-stroke depression: a placebo-
    controlled trial of antidepressants. Am J Psychiatry 2003;160(10):1823–9.
[13] de Groot M, Anderson R, Freedland KE, et al. Association of depression and diabetes
    complications: a meta-analysis. Psychosom Med 2001;63(4):619–30.
[14] Spiegel D, Giese-Davis J. Depression and cancer: mechanisms and disease progression.
    Biol Psychiatry 2003;54(3):269–82.

[15] Ganzini L, Smith DM, Fenn DS, et al. Depression and mortality in medically ill older adults. J Am Geriatr Soc 1997;45(3):307–12.
[16] Covinsky KE, Kahana E, Chin MH, et al. Depressive symptoms and 3-year mortality in older hospitalized medical patients. Ann Intern Med 1999;130(7):563–9.
[17] Rudisch B, Nemeroff CB. Epidemiology of comorbid coronary artery disease and depression. Biol Psychiatry 2003;54(3):227–40.
[18] Schleifer SJ, Macari-Hinson MM, Coyle DA, et al. The nature and course of depression following myocardial infarction. Arch Intern Med 1989;149(8):1785–9.
[19] Ziegelstein RC, Fauerbach JA, Stevens SS, et al. Patients with depression are less likely to follow recommendations to reduce cardiac risk during recovery from a myocardial infarction. Arch Intern Med 2000;160(12):1818–23.
[20] Lesperance F, Frasure-Smith N, Talajic M. Major depression before and after myocardial infarction: its nature and consequences. Psychosom Med 1996;58(2):99–110.
[21] Aben I, Verhey F, Strik J, et al. A comparative study into the one-year cumulative incidence of depression after stroke and myocardial infarction. J Neurol Neurosurg Psychiatry 2003;74(5):581–5.
[22] Carney RM, Rich MW, Tevelde A, et al. Major depressive disorder in coronary artery disease. Am J Cardiol 1987;60(16):1273–5.
[23] Dew MA, Roth LH, Schulberg HC, et al. Prevalence and predictors of depression and anxiety-related disorders during the year after heart transplantation. Gen Hosp Psychiatry 1996;18(6 Suppl):48S–61S.
[24] Jiang W, Alexander J, Christopher E, et al. Relationship of depression to increased risk of mortality and rehospitalization in patients with congestive heart failure. Arch Intern Med 2001;161(15):1849–56.
[25] Turvey CL, Schultz K, Arndt S, et al. Prevalence and correlates of depressive symptoms in a community sample of people suffering from heart failure. J Am Geriatr Soc 2002;50(12):2003–8.
[26] Mast BT, MacNeill SE, Lichtenberg PA. Post-stroke and clinically-defined vascular depression in geriatric rehabilitation patients. Am J Geriatr Psychiatry 2004;12(1):84–92.
[27] Rabkin JG, Charles E, Kass F. Hypertension and DSM-III depression in psychiatric outpatients. Am J Psychiatry 1983;140(8):1072–4.
[28] Bosworth HB, Bartash RM, Olsen MK, et al. The association of psychosocial factors and depression with hypertension among older adults. Int J Geriatr Psychiatry 2003;18(12):1142–8.
[29] Hamalainen J, Kaprio J, Isometsa E, et al. Cigarette smoking, alcohol intoxication and major depressive episode in a representative population sample. J Epidemiol Community Health 2001;55(8):573–6.
[30] Scarinci IC, Thomas J, Brantley PJ, et al. Examination of the temporal relationship between smoking and major depressive disorder among low-income women in public primary care clinics. Am J Health Promot 2002;16(6):323–30.
[31] Wulsin LR, Singal BM. Do depressive symptoms increase the risk for the onset of coronary disease? A systematic quantitative review. Psychosom Med 2003;65(2):201–10.
[32] Lesperance F, Frasure-Smith N, Talajic M, et al. Five-year risk of cardiac mortality in relation to initial severity and one-year changes in depression symptoms after myocardial infarction. Circulation 2002;105(9):1049–53.
[33] Robinson RG, Starr LB, Price TR. A two-year longitudinal study of mood disorders following stroke. Prevalence and duration at six months follow-up. Br J Psychiatry 1984;144:256–62.
[34] Astrom M, Adolfsson R, Asplund K. Major depression in stroke patients. A 3-year longitudinal study. Stroke 1993;24(7):976–82.
[35] Cassidy E, O'Connor R, O'Keane V. Prevalence of post-stroke depression in an Irish sample and its relationship with disability and outcome following inpatient rehabilitation. Disabil Rehabil 2004;26(2):71–7.

[36] Robinson RG. Poststroke depression: prevalence, diagnosis, treatment, and disease progression. Biol Psychiatry 2003;54(3):376–87.

[37] House A, Knapp P, Bamford J, et al. Mortality at 12 and 24 months after stroke may be associated with depressive symptoms at 1 month. Stroke 2001;32(3):696–701.

[38] Brown LC, Majumdar SR, Newman SC, et al. Type 2 diabetes does not increase risk of depression. CMAJ 2006;175(1):42–6.

[39] Sturm JW, Donnan GA, Dewey HM, et al. Quality of life after stroke: the North East Melbourne Stroke Incidence Study (NEMESIS). Stroke 2004;35(10):2340–5.

[40] Jonas BS, Franks P, Ingram DD. Are symptoms of anxiety and depression risk factors for hypertension? Longitudinal evidence from the National Health and Nutrition Examination Survey I Epidemiologic Follow-up Study. Arch Fam Med 1997;6:43–9.

[41] Davidson K, Jonas BS, Dixon KE, et al. Do depression symptoms predict early hypertension incidence in young adults in the CARDIA study? Coronary artery risk development in young adults. Arch Intern Med 2000;160:1495–500.

[42] Jess P, Eldrup J. The personality patterns in patients with duodenal ulcer and ulcer-like dyspepsia and their relationship to the course of the diseases. Hvidovre Ulcer Project Group. J Intern Med 1994;235(6):589–94.

[43] Levenstein S, Kaplan GA, Smith MW. Psychological predictors of peptic ulcer incidence in the Alameda County Study. J Clin Gastroenterol 1997;24(3):140–6.

[44] Gavard JA, Lustman PJ, Clouse RE. Prevalence of depression in adults with diabetes. An epidemiological evaluation. Diabetes Care 1993;16(8):1167–78.

[45] Anderson RJ, Freedland KE, Clouse RE, et al. The prevalence of comorbid depression in adults with diabetes: a meta-analysis. Diabetes Care 2001;24(6):1069–78.

[46] Brown LC, Majumdar SR, Newman SC, et al. History of depression increases risk of type 2 diabetes in younger adults. Diabetes Care 2005;28(5):1063–7.

[47] Katon W, von Korff M, Ciechanowski P, et al. Behavioral and clinical factors associated with depression among individuals with diabetes. Diabetes Care 2004;27(4):914–20.

[48] McDaniel JS, Musselman DL, Porter MR, et al. Depression in patients with cancer. Diagnosis, biology, and treatment. Arch Gen Psychiatry 1995;52:89–99.

[49] Brown KW, Levy AR, Rosberger Z, et al. Psychological distress and cancer survival: a follow-up 10 years after diagnosis. Psychosom Med 2003;65(4):636–43.

[50] Penninx BW, Guralnik JM, Pahor M, et al. Chronically depressed mood and cancer risk in older persons. J Natl Cancer Inst 1998;90(24):1888–93.

[51] Koenig HG, Meador KG, Cohen HJ, et al. Depression in elderly hospitalized patients with medical illness. Arch Intern Med 1988;148(9):1929–36.

[52] Koenig HG, Meador KG, Shelp F, et al. Major depressive disorder in hospitalized medically ill patients: an examination of young and elderly male veterans. J Am Geriatr Soc 1991;39(9):881–90.

[53] Wells KB, Rogers W, Burnam A, et al. How the medical comorbidity of depressed patients differs across health care settings: results from the Medical Outcomes Study. Am J Psychiatry 1991;148(12):1688–96.

[54] Patten SB. Long-term medical conditions and major depression in the Canadian population. Can J Psychiatry 1999;44(2):151–7.

[55] Watkins LL, Schneiderman N, Blumenthal JA, et al. ENRICHD Investigators. Cognitive and somatic symptoms of depression are associated with medical comorbidity in patients after acute myocardial infarction. Am Heart J 2003;146(1):48–54.

[56] Stein MB, Cox BJ, Afifi TO, et al. Does co-morbid depressive illness magnify the impact of chronic physical illness? A population-based perspective. Psychol Med 2006;36(5):587–96.

[57] Frasure-Smith N, Lesperance F, Prince RH, et al. Randomised trial of home-based psychosocial nursing intervention for patients recovering from myocardial infarction. Lancet 1997;350(9076):473–9.

[58] Nelson JC, Kennedy JS, Pollock BG, et al. Treatment of major depression with nortriptyline and paroxetine in patients with ischemic heart disease. Am J Psychiatry 1999;156(7): 1024–8.

[59] Strik JJ, Honig A, Lousberg R, et al. Efficacy and safety of fluoxetine in the treatment of patients with major depression after first myocardial infarction: findings from a double-blind, placebo-controlled trial. Psychosom Med 2000;62(6):783–9.

[60] Glassman AH, O'Connor CM, Califf RM, et al. Sertraline Antidepressant Heart Attack Randomized Trial (SADHART) Group. Sertraline treatment of major depression in patients with acute MI or unstable angina. JAMA 2002;288(6):701–9.

[61] Berkman LF, Blumenthal J, Burg M, et al. Enhancing Recovery in Coronary Heart Disease Patients Investigators (ENRICHD). Effects of treating depression and low perceived social support on clinical events after myocardial infarction: the Enhancing Recovery in Coronary Heart Disease Patients (ENRICHD) Randomized Trial. JAMA 2003;89(23):3106–16.

[62] Taylor CB, Youngblood ME, Catellier D, et al. ENRICHD Investigators. Effects of antidepressant medication on morbidity and mortality in depressed patients after myocardial infarction. Arch Gen Psychiatry 2005;62(7):792–8.

[63] Andersen G, Vestergaard K, Lauritzen L. Effective treatment of post-stroke depression with the selective serotonin reuptake inhibitor citalopram. Stroke 1994;25(6):1099–104.

[64] Robinson RG, Schultz SK, Castillo C, et al. Nortriptyline versus fluoxetine in the treatment of depression and in short-term recovery after stroke: a placebo-controlled, double-blind study. Am J Psychiatry 2000;157(3):351–9.

[65] Wiart L, Petit H, Joseph PA, et al. Fluoxetine in early post-stroke depression: a double-blind placebo-controlled study. Stroke 2000;31(8):1829–32.

[66] Fruehwald S, Gatterbauer E, Rehak P, et al. Early fluoxetine treatment of post-stroke depression—a three-month double-blind placebo-controlled study with an open-label long-term follow up. J Neurol 2003;250(3):347–51.

[67] Choi-Kwon S, Han SW, Kwon SU, et al. Fluoxetine treatment in poststroke depression, emotional incontinence, and anger proneness: a double-blind, placebo-controlled study. Stroke 2006;37(1):156–61.

[68] Narushima K, Kosier JT, Robinson RG. Preventing poststroke depression: a 12-week double-blind randomized treatment trial and 21-month follow-up. J Nerv Ment Dis 2002; 190(5):296–303.

[69] Almeida OP, Waterreus A, Hankey GJ. Preventing depression after stroke: results from a randomized placebo-controlled trial. J Clin Psychiatry 2006;67(7):1104–9.

[70] Goodnick PJ. Use of antidepressants in treatment of comorbid diabetes mellitus and depression as well as in diabetic neuropathy. Ann Clin Psychiatry 2001;13(1):31–41.

[71] Lustman PJ, Griffith LS, Clouse RE, et al. Effects of nortriptyline on depression and glycemic control in diabetes: results of a double-blind, placebo-controlled trial. Psychosom Med 1997;59(3):241–50.

[72] Lustman PJ, Freedland KE, Griffith LS, et al. Fluoxetine for depression in diabetes: a randomized double-blind placebo-controlled trial. Diabetes Care 2000;23(5):618–23.

[73] Lustman PJ, Griffith LS, Freedland KE, et al. Cognitive behavior therapy for depression in type 2 diabetes mellitus. A randomized, controlled trial. Ann Intern Med 1998;129(8): 613–21.

[74] Katon WJ, Von Korff M, Lin EH, et al. The Pathways Study: a randomized trial of collaborative care in patients with diabetes and depression. Arch Gen Psychiatry 2004;61(10): 1042–9.

[75] Williams S, Dale J. The effectiveness of treatment for depression/depressive symptoms in adults with cancer: a systematic review. Br J Cancer 2006;94(3):372–90.

[76] van Heeringen K, Zivkov M. Pharmacological treatment of depression in cancer patients. A placebo-controlled study of mianserin. Br J Psychiatry 1996;169(4):440–3.

[77] Razavi D, Allilaire JF, Smith M, et al. The effect of fluoxetine on anxiety and depression symptoms in cancer patients. Acta Psychiatr Scand 1996;94:205–10.

[78] Morrow GR, Hickok JT, Roscoe JA, et al. Differential effects of paroxetine on fatigue and depression: a randomized double-blind trial from the University of Rochester Cancer Centre Community Clinical Oncology Program. J Clin Oncol 2003;21:4635–41.

[79] Roscoe JA, Morrow GR, Hickok JT, et al. Effect of paroxetine hydrochloride (Paxil) on fatigue and depression in breast cancer patients receiving chemotherapy. Breast Cancer Res Treat 2005;89:243–9.

[80] Holland JC, Romano SJ, Heiligenstein JH, et al. A controlled trial of fluoxetine and desipramine in depressed women with advanced cancer. Psychooncology 1998;7:291–300.

[81] Pezzella G, Moslinger-Gehmayr R, Contu A. Treatment of depression in patients with breast cancer: a comparison between paroxetine and amitriptyline. Breast Cancer Res Treat 2001;70:1–10.

[82] Ash G, Dickens CM, Creed FH, et al. The effects of dothiepin on subjects with rheumatoid arthritis and depression. Rheumatology (Oxford) 1999;38(10):959–67.

[83] Bird H, Broggini M. Paroxetine versus amitriptyline for treatment of depression associated with rheumatoid arthritis: a randomized, double blind, parallel group study. J Rheumatol 2000;27(12):2791–7.

[84] Parker JC, Smarr KL, Slaughter JR, et al. Management of depression in rheumatoid arthritis: a combined pharmacologic and cognitive-behavioral approach. Arthritis Rheum 2003;49(6):766–77.

[85] Popkin MK, Callies AL, Mackenzie TB. The outcome of antidepressant use in the medically ill. Arch Gen Psychiatry 1985;42:1160–3.

[86] Koenig HG, Goli V, Shelp F, et al. Antidepressant use in elderly medical inpatients: lessons from an attempted clinical trial. J Gen Intern Med 1989;4(6):498–505.

[87] Keitner GI, Ryan CE, Miller IW, et al. 12-month outcome of patients with major depression and comorbid psychiatric or medical illness (compound depression). Am J Psychiatry 1991;148(3):345–50.

[88] Small GW, Birkett M, Meyers BS, et al. Impact of physical illness on quality of life and antidepressant response in geriatric major depression: Fluoxetine Collaborative Study Group. J Am Geriatr Soc 1996;44:1220–5.

[89] Evans M, Hammond M, Wilson K, et al. Placebo-controlled treatment trial of depression in elderly physically ill patients. Int J Geriatr Psychiatry 1997;12(8):817–24.

[90] Evans M, Hammond M, Wilson K, et al. Treatment of depression in the elderly: effect of physical illness on response. Int J Geriatr Psychiatry 1997;12(12):1189–94.

[91] Koike AK, Unutzer J, Wells KB. Improving the care for depression in patients with comorbid medical illness. Am J Psychiatry 2002;159(10):1738–45.

[92] Oslin DW, Datto CJ, Kallan MJ, et al. Association between medical comorbidity and treatment outcomes in late-life depression. J Am Geriatr Soc 2002;50(5):823–8.

[93] Papakostas GI, Petersen T, Iosifescu DV, et al. Axis III disorders in treatment-resistant major depressive disorder. Psychiatry Res 2003;118(2):183–8.

[94] Iosifescu DV, Nierenberg AA, Alpert JE, et al. The impact of medical comorbidity on acute treatment in major depressive disorder. Am J Psychiatry 2003;160(12):2122–7.

[95] Perlis RH, Iosifescu DV, Alpert JE, et al. Medical comorbidity does not moderate response to augmentation or dose increase among depressed outpatients resistant to fluoxetine 20 mg/day. Psychosomatics 2004;45(3):224–9.

[96] Alexopoulos GS, Meyers BS, Robert YC, et al. Executive dysfunction and long-term outcomes of geriatric depression. Arch Gen Psychiatry 2000;57(3):285–90.

[97] Iosifescu DV, Nierenberg AA, Alpert JE, et al. Comorbid medical illness and relapse of major depressive disorder in the continuation phase of treatment. Psychosomatics 2004;45:419–25.

[98] Simon GE, Von Korff M, Lin E. Clinical and functional outcomes of depression treatment in patients with and without chronic medical illness. Psychol Med 2005;35(2):271–9.

[99] Bogner HR, Cary MS, Bruce ML, et al. The role of medical comorbidity in outcome of major depression in primary care: the PROSPECT study. Am J Geriatr Psychiatry 2005;13(10): 861–8.

[100] Harpole LH, Williams JW Jr, Olsen MK, et al. Improving depression outcomes in older adults with comorbid medical illness. Gen Hosp Psychiatry 2005;27(1):4–12.

[101] Ciechanowski PS, Katon WJ, Russo JE. Depression and diabetes: impact of depressive symptoms on adherence, function, and costs. Arch Intern Med 2000;160(21): 3278–85.

[102] DeVane CL. Metabolism and pharmacokinetics of selective serotonin reuptake inhibitors. Cell Mol Neurobiol 1999;19(4):443–66.

[103] Brown ES, Varghese FP, McEwen BS. Association of depression with medical illness: does cortisol play a role? Biol Psychiatry 2004;55(1):1–9.

[104] Arana GW, Baldessarini JR, Ornsteen M. The dexamethasone suppression test for diagnosis and prognosis in psychiatry. Arch Gen Psychiatry 1985;42:1193–204.

[105] Lenox RH, Teyser JM, Rothschild B, et al. Failure to normalize the dexamethasone suppression test: association with length of illness. Biol Psychiatry 1985;20: 329–52.

[106] Targum SD. Persistent neuroendocrine dysregulation in major depressive disorder: a marker for early relapse. Biol Psychiatry 1984;19(3):305–18.

[107] Young EA, Lopez JF, Murphy-Weinberg V, et al. Hormonal evidence for altered responsiveness to social stress in major depression. Neuropsychopharmacology 2000;23(4): 411–8.

[108] McEwen BS. Effects of adverse experiences for brain structure and function. Biol Psychiatry 2000;48(8):721–31.

[109] Sheline YI, Wang PW, Gado MH, et al. Hippocampal atrophy in recurrent major depression. Proc Natl Acad Sci U S A 1996;93(9):3908–13.

[110] Steffens DC, Byrum CE, McQuoid DR, et al. Hippocampal volume in geriatric depression. Biol Psychiatry 2000;48:301–9.

[111] Krakoff LR. Glucocorticoid excess syndromes causing hypertension. Cardiol Clin 1988; 6(4):537–45.

[112] Lechin F, van der Dijs B, Rada I, et al. Plasma neurotransmitters and cortisol in duodenal ulcer patients. Role of stress. Dig Dis Sci 1990;35(11):1313–9.

[113] Roy MS, Roy A, Brown S. Increased urinary-free cortisol outputs in diabetic patients. J Diabetes Complications 1998;12(1):24–7.

[114] Hricik DE, Mayes JT, Schulak JA. Independent effects of cyclosporine and prednisone on posttransplant hypercholesterolemia. Am J Kidney Dis 1991;18(3):353–8.

[115] Dunn AJ, Swiergiel AH, de Beaurepaire R. Cytokines as mediators of depression: what can we learn from animal studies? Neurosci Biobehav Rev 2005;29(4–5): 891–909.

[116] Gottsater A, Forsblad J, Matzsch T, et al. Interleukin-1 receptor antagonist is detectable in human carotid artery plaques and is related to triglyceride levels and Chlamydia pneumoniae IgA antibodies. J Intern Med 2002;251(1):61–8.

[117] Stenvinkel P, Heimburger O, Jogestrand T. Elevated interleukin-6 predicts progressive carotid artery atherosclerosis in dialysis patients: association with Chlamydia pneumoniae seropositivity. Am J Kidney Dis 2002;39(2):274–82.

[118] Cottone S, Mule G, Amato F, et al. Amplified biochemical activation of endothelial function in hypertension associated with moderate to severe renal failure. J Nephrol 2002;15(6): 643–8.

[119] van der Meer IM, de Maat MP, Bots ML, et al. Inflammatory mediators and cell adhesion molecules as indicators of severity of atherosclerosis: the Rotterdam Study. Arterioscler Thromb Vasc Biol 2002;22(5):838–42.

[120] Reid PT, Sallenave JM. Cytokines in the pathogenesis of chronic obstructive pulmonary disease. Curr Pharm Des 2003;9(1):25–38.

[121] Woodman RJ, Watts GF, Puddey IB, et al. Leukocyte count and vascular function in type 2 diabetic subjects with treated hypertension. Atherosclerosis 2002;163(1): 175–81.

[122] Yirmiya R, Pollak Y, Morag M, et al. Illness, cytokines, and depression. Ann N Y Acad Sci 2000;917:478–87.

[123] Meyers CA. Mood and cognitive disorders in cancer patients receiving cytokine therapy. In: Dantzer R, Wollman EE, Yirmiya R, editors. Cytokines, stress and depression. New York: Kluwer Academic/Plenum Publishers; 1999. p. 75–81.

[124] Dantzer R, Wollman E, Vitkovic L, et al. Cytokines and depression: fortuitous or causative association. Mol Psychiatry 1999;4(4):328–32.

[125] Dantzer R. Cytokine-induced sickness behavior: where do we stand? Brain Behav Immun 2001;15(1):7–24.

Brain Correlates of Antidepressant Treatment Outcome from Neuroimaging Studies in Depression

Darin D. Dougherty, MD[a],*, Scott L. Rauch, MD[b]

[a]Department of Psychiatry, Massachusetts General Hospital,
15 Parkman Street, Boston, MA 02114, USA
[b]Department of Psychiatry, McLean Hospital, 116 Mill Street, Belmont, MA 02478, USA

Psychiatric research, including postmortem and neuroimaging studies, has contributed a great deal to the understanding of the pathophysiology of major depressive disorder (MDD). The ultimate goal of this psychiatric research is better diagnosis and treatment of individuals who have MDD. In this context, a growing number of neuroimaging studies have focused on correlates of treatment response. This review begins by reviewing findings from psychiatric research involving subjects who have major depression. It then discusses general issues involved in conducting neuroimaging studies that seek to identify correlates of treatment response. It concludes with a review of neuroimaging studies of treatment response in depression and integrates these findings into current models regarding the pathophysiology of major depression.

NEUROIMAGING STUDIES OF MAJOR DEPRESSION

An integrated cortical-limbic network is implicated in normal affective processing and in the pathophysiology of mood disorders [1–6]. Structures in this network interact with one another extensively, including contributing to cortico-thalamo-striatal circuits that seem to be related importantly to both affective and cognitive processing. This article reviews neuroimaging studies in mood disorders, focusing on key elements of these circuits. Converging data implicate the previously mentioned network of brain regions in the pathophysiology of major depressive episodes, regardless of whether they occur in the context of unipolar major depression or bipolar disorder.

Prefrontal Cortex and Anterior Paralimbic Regions

The prefrontal cortex (PFC) is not a monolithic entity; there are multiple subregions associated with discrete functions. In general, however, PFC function can be divided into two broad categories: (1) working memory-executive function-attention, and (2) the coupling of thoughts, memories, and experience

*Corresponding author. E-mail address: ddougherty@partners.org (D.D. Dougherty).

0193-953X/07/$ – see front matter
doi:10.1016/j.psc.2006.12.007

with corresponding emotional and visceral states. Dorsolateral PFC (DLPFC) and dorsal regions of the medial PFC (including the dorsal anterior cingulate cortex [ACC]) are involved in working memory-executive function-attention. Cognitive activation paradigms in healthy volunteers have shown DLPFC involvement in tasks of working memory, in encoding and retrieval processes in episodic memory tasks, and in tasks of forward planning and problem solving [7–9]. DLPFC activations during working and episodic memory tasks reflect the use of executive control processes such as monitoring, updating, and manipulating information held in working memory [7–9]. These processes contribute to a variety of complex cognitive skills including the ability to organize information during learning (encoding) as well as forward planning and problem solving. Converging data indicate that the dorsal ACC, also referred to as the "cognitive division" of the ACC, is involved in cognition and motor control. For example, in functional neuroimaging studies the dorsal ACC has been activated by tasks that involve target and motor response selection [10–14], error detection and performance monitoring [15,16], novelty detection [17], competition monitoring [18–20], motivational valence assignment [21], and reward-based decision making [22]. In contrast, ventral regions of the medial PFC (including more ventral regions of the ACC), orbitofrontal cortex, and subgenual PFC are involved in the coupling of thoughts, memories, and experience with corresponding emotional and visceral states. These regions are often referred to as "paralimbic" regions (other paralimbic regions include the insula and temporal pole) and play an important role in linking cognition with visceral states and emotion. All these regions have been associated with the production of emotional states and behavior [23,24] and are believed to be involved in the mediation of associated autonomic activity.

Structural abnormalities in mood disorders have been detected in postmortem studies and morphometric MRI studies (for reviews see Refs. [25–28]). Structural abnormalities have been found in studies of patients who have mood disorders in a number of subregions of the PFC, including volumetric reductions in the DLPFC [29,30] and regions of the ventral PFC, including the orbitofrontal cortex [30,31] and subgenual PFC [32]. Neutral-condition (ie, resting or continuous performance task, as opposed to more complex task-activated conditions) functional neuroimaging studies of patients who have affective disorders consistently have found functional abnormalities in the PFC, usually in the left hemisphere (for reviews see Refs. [1,2,5,6,27,28,33]). Specifically, numerous neutral-condition functional neuroimaging studies have demonstrated decreased regional cerebral blood flow (rCBF) and glucose metabolism in DLPFC and subgenual PFC and increased rCBF and glucose metabolism in orbitofrontal cortex in patients during major depressive episodes. In addition, functional neuroimaging studies using activation paradigms in patients who have affective disorders have demonstrated abnormalities of left PFC regions, particularly inferior frontal regions, during both emotion induction and cognitive tasks when compared with control subjects [34–42].

ACC differences have been less consistent than those found in other PFC regions in patients who have mood disorder. Decreased activity in the PFC ventral to the genu of the corpus callosum (subgenual) was observed both in depressed patients who had familial bipolar disorder and in depressed patients who had familial MDD [3]. Decreased subgenual PFC cortical activity was accompanied by volume reductions in gray matter [3,43]. One study, however, noted that depressed patients who had nonfamilial MDD had increased subgenual PFC cortical activity when compared with healthy controls [44]. In a combined sample of patients who had bipolar disorder or unipolar major depression, Hamilton Depression Scale scores correlated directly with right ACC metabolism, and Spielberger Anxiety-State Scale scores correlated directly with left ACC metabolism [45]. There has been considerable variability in ACC/medial PFC activity in studies of patients who have unipolar major depression. Thus, patients who have unipolar major depression have been reported to have decreased [3,46–58], unchanged [6,59–73], or increased [44,74] ACC activity.

Taken together, these studies strongly suggest that multiple subregions of the PFC are involved in the pathophysiology of mood disorders. Metabolic differences between depressed patients and controls have been more consistent in the subgenual PFC and DLPFC than in the ACC.

Medial Temporal Lobes

The medial temporal lobes include the hippocampal and amygdala regions. The hippocampus is crucial for learning because it is the central brain region responsible for explicit, declarative, and episodic memory. The amygdala is central to assigning emotional valence to sensory stimuli and also plays a role in learning. Emotional valence is associated with intrinsic properties of the stimulus and with memories associated with the particular stimulus. Therefore, the hippocampus and amygdala work in concert in identifying the emotional significance of environmental stimuli and the production of affective states.

Both morphometric MRI and postmortem studies of the medial temporal lobe in cohorts of mood-disordered subjects have shown increased amygdala volume [75–80] and decreased hippocampal volume [77,78,81]. Neutral-condition functional neuroimaging studies have demonstrated decreased glucose metabolism in the hippocampus in depressed cohorts and have found a negative correlation between glucose metabolism in the hippocampus and depression severity [72]. Additionally, a growing number of neutral-condition functional neuroimaging studies have demonstrated increased rCBF and glucose metabolism in the amygdala in depressed cohorts [51,74,82–86] with the majority implicating the left, rather than the right, amygdala. These findings are consistent with functional neuroimaging studies using emotion-induction methods that have found increased left amygdala activity during sadness induction in healthy volunteers [87–89]. Functional MRI (fMRI) studies of adult depressed patients during presentation of emotional facial expressions have demonstrated left amygdala hyperresponsivity [90–92] and have found that this exaggerated amygdala activation returns toward normal with successful antidepressant treatment [90,91]. Consistent with this literature, another fMRI study demonstrated that adult depressed patients have sustained amygdala response to negative words when compared with control subjects [93]. Finally, depressed patients who later respond to sleep deprivation had baseline increased left amygdala rCMR in one study [94] and right hippocampal-amygdala complex rCBF in another [95]. Taken together, these data suggest that the medial temporal lobe is involved in the pathophysiology of mood disorders, with decreases in volume and function of the hippocampus and increases in volume and pathologic activation of the amygdala noted in patients who have mood disorders (for reviews see Refs. [1,96,97]).

TREATMENT-RESPONSE PARADIGMS IN NEUROIMAGING RESEARCH

Neuroimaging studies of correlates of treatment response can contribute to an understanding of pathophysiology and perhaps provide predictors of treatment response while offering clues to the mechanism of effective therapies. These studies involve collecting pretreatment imaging data that are analyzed subsequently in light of clinical response. Response may be characterized categorically (responders versus nonresponders) or as a continuous variable based on clinical rating scale results. A number of general issues must be considered when designing or interpreting the results of this type of study [98,99].

Phenotyping and Clinical Trial Design

There are many clinical characteristics of major depression that must be controlled for in any neuroimaging studies of this population. Differences in clinical presentation may correspond with differences in changes in brain function. For example, studies of depressed patients may include subjects who have unipolar depression or bipolar depression, subjects who have different subtypes of depression (eg, atypical depression or melancholic depression, subjects with or without psychotic features, and subjects with single episode versus recurrent episodes). Even if these variables are controlled for, there still may be significant heterogeneity between individuals diagnosed with major depression. Because the diagnosis of a major depressive episode relies on the presence of at least five of nine symptoms listed in the *Diagnostic and Statistical Manual for Mental Disorders*, edition 4, it is possible that two subjects, each diagnosed with depression, may share only one common clinical symptom. Many patients who have major depression also suffer from comorbid illnesses (both psychiatric and medical) that may confound results. In addition, concurrent pharmacotherapy, psychotherapy, or other therapeutic interventions can confound results of neuroimaging studies evaluating treatment response. Therefore, the careful phenotyping of subjects, selecting subjects within as narrow a diagnostic category as possible, and minimizing comorbid illness and concurrent treatment will all maximize the interpretability of the study results.

The tools used for clinical phenotyping are crucial as well. Using standardized clinical interview tools to determine diagnosis is preferable to a chart review, for example. In addition, the choice of outcome measure may affect the quality of the data drastically. The use of standard outcome measures for depression (such as the Hamilton Depression Scale and Beck Depression Inventory) will provide better-quality data than a simple Likert scale. The method of administering the scales and the intervals between assessments should be the same for all subjects. Ideally, for all subjects the type of treatment, the amount of treatment (eg, medication dosage), and duration of treatment acquisition of baseline imaging data should be identical. If there is variance for any of these factors, these issues must be addressed statistically.

Data Acquisition and Analysis

The majority of neuroimaging studies of correlates of treatment response have employed neutral-state paradigms in which subjects are studied during a nominal resting state. Fluorodeoxyglucose positron emission tomography, which measures resting cerebral glucose metabolism, typically has been used for such studies. Neuroimaging studies that use activation paradigms could be used also. In addition, other neuroimaging modalities such as structural neuroimaging, other functional neuroimaging modalities (eg, fMRI), neuroreceptor imaging, and magnetic resonance spectroscopy could be used also. Although this review focuses on neuroimaging studies of correlates of treatment response, acquiring imaging data again following treatment (pretreatment/posttreatment design) may be particularly informative regarding the mechanisms of action of therapeutic interventions.

The clinical outcome data from a neuroimaging study of correlates of treatment response typically are analyzed using one of two methods. One method involves a categorical approach in which subjects are categorized as responders or nonresponders following the clinical trial. In this case, constructing group images from the imaging data and comparing the group images of the responders with those of the nonresponders may provide information regarding features that differentiate responders from nonresponders. The other method uses covariate analyses of changes in clinical rating scale data. The use of continuous measures may elucidate more subtle predictors of response than analyses by categorical designation (eg, responders or nonresponders). In addition, the use of continuous measures obviates the need for an arbitrary definition of "responder." Testing for confounding mediating variables is important, however, because imaging data may seem to correlate with clinical response but actually correlate with another variable either partially involved or not involved in clinical response if this analysis method is used.

Finally, two approaches to analysis of the imaging data typically are used. The first, voxel-wise analysis, uses statistical parametric mapping in which statistical analyses are conducted in a voxel-by-voxel manner for the entire brain. In contrast, region-of-interest (ROI) approaches test hypotheses for predetermined anatomical regions. The ROI approach allows hypothesis testing of precise anatomic ROIs. The ROI approach, however, may fail to detect significant results outside the predetermined ROIs, and effects within a ROI may not be detected because of dilution resulting from only a subterritory of the ROI correlating with subsequent treatment response.

STUDIES OF CORRELATES BETWEEN NEUROIMAGING FINDINGS AND TREATMENT RESPONSE IN SUBJECTS WHO HAVE MAJOR DEPRESSION

Again, neuroimaging studies designed to identify predictors of response in patients who have unipolar major depression involve acquiring neuroimaging data from subjects at baseline (before initiating treatment). The subjects then undergo treatment, and analytical methods are used to determine correlations between the baseline imaging data and subsequent clinical response.

Numerous studies have shown that patients who exhibit increased ACC activity exhibit superior subsequent response to sleep deprivation, an intervention known to provide transient relief from depressive symptoms in many patients [94,95,100–102]. This finding of increased baseline ACC activity correlating with subsequent treatment response is consistent in studies of neuroimaging correlates of treatment response following treatment with medications as well [5,103,104]. Other neutral-condition studies have found that higher metabolism in the left gyrus rectus [68] and lower metabolism in the medial PFC [105] correlated with response to medication.

The consistent finding of baseline ACC activity predicting subsequent treatment response is intriguing given current models of the pathophysiology of MDD. As described previously, there is substantial evidence that cortical-limbic networks are central to the pathophysiology of major depression. One synthesis of these data notes that dorsal cortical-limbic structures exhibit decreased activity at rest, and ventral cortical-limbic structures exhibit increased activity at rest in patients who have major depression [5]. This model posits that the pregenual ACC plays a crucial role in integrating normal function between these dorsal and ventral "compartments." The bulk of the neutral-condition studies of neuroimaging correlates of treatment response suggest that higher baseline activity in the ACC correlates with subsequent treatment response. This finding suggests that the healthy functioning of the ACC, particularly the pregenual ACC region that is so important for communication between the diseased dorsal and ventral compartments, is a necessary neural substrate for treatment response in depressed individuals. The fact that the variability in function of this territory at baseline may account for the degree of treatment response likely also accounts for the inconsistent findings regarding the role of the ACC in the pathophysiology of MDD.

Although the majority of neuroimaging studies of correlates of treatment response have used neutral-condition paradigms, two studies have used activation paradigms. One study found that increased ACC activation in response to viewing negative pictures correlated with symptom reduction following treatment with venlafaxine [35]. The other found that increased bilateral amygdalar activation in response to viewing emotional faces predicted response to antidepressants [106]. These studies point to the potential usefulness of activation paradigms in neuroimaging studies of correlates of treatment response; future studies using neuroreceptor imaging and magnetic resonance spectroscopy may prove useful also.

Although studies examining neuroimaging correlates of treatment response may be informative regarding the baseline neural substrates required for treatment response, most have little potential for clinical usefulness because of the high cost of the imaging studies compared with the relatively low

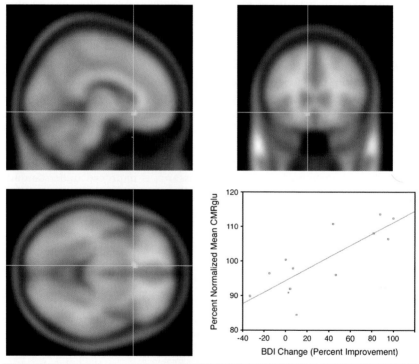

Fig. 1. Positron emission tomography/MRI superimposition, three views (sagittal, coronal, axial). Z-score maps demonstrating the principal finding of a statistically significant correlation between preoperative regional cerebral metabolic rate of glucose within left subgenual prefrontal cortex and Beck Depression Inventory improvement following anterior cingulotomy. The upper panels and the lower left panel show the locus in brain of significant correlation, as viewed from the three conventional orthogonal perspectives. The intersection of the crosshairs corresponds to the site of peak correlation (z score = 3.32; MNI coordinates = −8, 24, −8); this site defines the voxel of peak statistical significance used to generate the data depicted graphically (*lower right panel*). Specifically, for this voxel, the Pearson product moment correlation between rCMRglu and BDI improvement yielded $r^2(11) = .81$, $P = .001$. (*From:* Dougherty DD, Weiss AP, Cosgrove GR, et al. Cerebral metabolic correlates as potential predictors of response to anterior cingulotomy for major depression. J Neurosurg 2003;99:1012; with permission.)

cost of the therapeutic intervention. Any test that may predict outcome for higher-cost and/or higher-risk interventions may prove ultimately to be clinical useful, however. For example, ablative limbic system surgery techniques such as anterior cingulotomy are used for patients who have treatment-refractory MDD and obsessive-compulsive disorder. In one study of 13 patients who had treatment-refractory MDD undergoing anterior cingulotomy, pretreatment metabolism in the left subgenual PFC and left thalamus correlated with subsequent treatment response [107]. Although these findings are distinct from other studies that suggest that baseline pregenual ACC function is crucial for response to other antidepressant therapies, these subjects were markedly more ill than those in the other studies. Also, other neural substrates may be important in treatment response following ablative limbic system surgery (Fig. 1).

SUMMARY

Although neutral-state functional neuroimaging studies have improved the understanding of the pathophysiology of major depression, studies that employ state manipulations may provide further information. Such interventions may include cognitive activation or symptom provocation paradigms or studies of the effects of acute or chronic pharmacologic treatment. This article has reviewed issues surrounding functional neuroimaging studies of treatment. Because the ultimate goal of psychiatric research is improved understanding of the pathophysiology as well as treatment of mental illness, the proposed contribution of these studies is the development of tests that will guide case management and thus be clinically useful.

References

[1] Davidson RJ, Pizzagalli D, Nitschke JB, et al. Depression: perspectives from affective neuroscience. Annu Rev Psychol 2002;53:545–74.

[2] Dougherty DD, Rauch SL. Neuroimaging and neurobiological models of depression. Harv Rev Psychiatry 1997;5:138–59.

[3] Drevets WC, Price JL, Simpson JR Jr, et al. Subgenual prefrontal cortex abnormalities in mood disorders. Nature 1997;386(6627):824–7.

[4] Ketter TA, Wang PW, Dieckmann N, et al. Brain anatomic circuits and the pathophysiology of affective disorders. In: Soares J, editor. Brain imaging in affective disorders. New York: Marcel-Dekker; 2002. p. 611–26.

[5] Mayberg HS. Limbic-cortical dysregulation: a proposed model of depression. J Neuropsychiatry Clin Neurosci 1997;9:471–81.

[6] Videbach P. PET measurements of brain glucose metabolism and blood flow in major depressive disorder: a critical review. Acta Psychiatr Scand 2001;101: 11–20.

[7] Owen AM, Evans AC, Petrides M. Evidence for a two-stage model of spatial working memory processing within the lateral frontal cotex: a positron emission tomography study. Cereb Cortex 1996;8:353–64.

[8] D'Esposito M, Aguirre GK, Zarahn E, et al. Functional MRI studies of spatial and nonspatial working memory. Brain Res Cogn Brain Res 1998;7:1–13.

[9] Smith EE, Jonides J. Storage and executive processes in the frontal lobes. Science 1999;283:1657–61.

[10] Posner MI, Petersen SE, Fox PT, et al. Localization of cognitive operations in the human brain. Science 1988;240(4859):1627–31.

[11] Frith CD, Friston KJ, Liddle PF, et al. Willed action and the prefrontal cortex in man: a study with PET. Proc R Soc Lond B Biol Sci 1991;244:241–6.

[12] Paus T, Petrides M, Evans AC, et al. Role of the human anterior cingulate cortex in the control of oculomotor, manual, and speech responses: a positron emission tomography study. J Neurophysiol 1993;70(2):453–69.

[13] Badgaiyan RD, Posner MI. Mapping the cingulate cortex in response selection and monitoring. Neuroimage 1998;7:255–60.

[14] Turken AU, Swick D. Response selection in the human anterior cingulate cortex. Nat Neurosci 1999;2:920–4.

[15] Gehring WJ, Knight RT. Prefrontal-cingulate interactions in action monitoring. Nat Neurosci 2000;3:516–20.

[16] Luu P, Flaisch T, Tucker DM. Medial frontal cortex in action monitoring. J Neurosci 2000;20:464–9.

[17] Clark VP, Fannon S, Lai S, et al. Responses to rare visual target and distractor stimuli using event-related fMRI. J Neurophysiol 2000;83(5):3133–9.

[18] Carter CS, Braver TS, Barch DM, et al. Anterior cingulate cortex, error detection, and the online monitoring of performance. Science 1998;280(5364):747–9.

[19] Botvinic M, Nystrom LE, Fissell K, et al. Conflict monitoring versus selection- for-action in anterior cingulate cortex. Nature 1999;402(6758):179–81.

[20] Carter CS, Macdonald AM, Botvinick M, et al. Parsing executive processes: strategic vs. evaluative functions of the anterior cingulate cortex. Proc Natl Acad Sci U S A 2000;97(4):1944–8.

[21] Mesulam MM. Large-scale neurocognitive networks and distributed processing for attention, language and memory. Ann Neurol 1990;28:597–613.

[22] Bush G, Vogt BA, Holmes J, et al. Dorsal anterior cingulate cortex: a role in reward-based decision making. Proc Natl Acad Sci U S A 2002;99(1):523–8.

[23] Bush G, Luu P, Posner MI. Cognitive and emotional influences in anterior cingulate cortex. Trends Cogn Sci 2000;4(6):215–22.

[24] Phillips ML, Drevets WC, Rauch SL, et al. Neurobiology of emotion perception I: the neural basis of normal emotion perception. Biol Psychiatry 2003;54(5):504–14.

[25] Beardon CE, Hoffman KM, Cannon TD. The neuropsychology and neuroanatomy of bipolar affective disorder: a critical review. Bipolar Disord 2001;3:106–50.

[26] Harrison PJ. The neuropathology of primary mood disorder. Brain 2002;125:1428–49.

[27] Sheline YI. Neuroimaging studies of mood disorder effects on the brain. Biol Psychiatry 2003;54:338–52.

[28] Strakowski SM, DelBello MP, Adler C, et al. Neuroimaging in bipolar disorder. Bipolar Disord 2000;2:148–64.

[29] Cotter D, Mackay D, Chana G, et al. Reduced neuronal size and glial cell density in area 9 of the dorsolateral prefrontal cortex in subjects with major depressive disorder. Cereb Cortex 2002;12:386–94.

[30] Rajkowska G, Miguel-Hidalgo JJ, Wei J, et al. Morphometric evidence for neuronal and glial prefrontal cell pathology in major depression. Biol Psychiatry 1999;45:1085–98.

[31] Bremner JD, Vythilingam M, Vermetten E, et al. Reduced volume of orbitofrontal cortex in major depression. Biol Psychiatry 2002;51:273–9.

[32] Ongur D, Drevets WC, Price JL. Glial reduction in the subgenual prefrontal cortex in mood disorders. Proc Natl Acad Sci U S A 1998;95:13290–5.

[33] Drevets WC. Neuroimaging studies of mood disorders. Biol Psychiatry 2000;48:813–29.

[34] Blumberg HP, Leung HC, Skudlarski P, et al. A functional magnetic resonance imaging study of bipolar disorder: state- and trait-related dysfunction in ventral prefrontal cortices. Arch Gen Psychiatry 2003;60:601–9.

[35] Davidson RJ, Irwin W, Anderle MJ, et al. The neural substrates of affective processing in depressed patients treated with venlafaxine. Am J Psychiatry 2003;160:64–75.

[36] Dougherty DD, Rauch SL, Deckersbach T, et al. Ventromedial prefrontal cortex and amygdala dysfunction during an anger induction positron emission tomography study in patients with major depressive disorder with anger attacks. Arch Gen Psychiatry 2004;61: 795–804.

[37] Elliott R, Baker SC, Rogers RD, et al. Prefrontal dysfunction in depressed patients performing a complex planning task: a study using positron emission tomography. Psychol Med 1997;27:931–42.

[38] Elliott R, Sahakian BJ, Michael A, et al. Abnormal neural response to feedback on planning and guessing tasks in patients with unipolar depression. Psychol Med 1998;28:559–71.

[39] Elliott R, Rubinsztein JS, Sahakian BJ, et al. The neural basis of mood-congruent processing biases in depression. Arch Gen Psychiatry 2002;59:597–604.

[40] Kumari V, Mitterschiffthaler MT, Teasdale JD, et al. Neural abnormalities during cognitive generation of affect in treatment-resistant depression. Biol Psychol 2003;54:777–91.

[41] Liotti M, Mayberg HS, McGinnis S, et al. Unmasking disease-specific cerebral blood flow abnormalities: mood challenge in patients with remitted unipolar depression. Am J Psychiatry 2002;159:1830–40.

[42] Mitterschiffthaler MT, Kumari V, Malhi GS, et al. Neural response to pleasant stimuli in anhedonia: an fMRI study. Neuroreport 2003;14:177–82.

[43] Hirayasu Y, Shenton ME, Salisbury DF, et al. Subgenual cingulate cortex volume in first-episode psychosis. Am J Psychiatry 1999;156(7):1091–3.

[44] Videbech P, Ravnkilde B, Pedersen TH, et al. The Danish PET/depression project: clinical symptoms and cerebral blood flow. A regions-of-interest analysis. Acta Psychiatr Scand 2002;106(1):35–44.

[45] Osuch EA, Ketter TA, Kimbrell TA, et al. Regional cerebral metabolism associated with anxiety symptoms in affective disorder patients. Biol Psychiatry 2000;48(10):1020–3.

[46] Hagman JO, Buchsbaum MS, Wu JC, et al. Comparison of regional brain metabolism in bulimia nervosa and affective disorder assessed with positron emission tomography. J Affect Disord 1990;19(3):153–62.

[47] Hurwitz TA, Clark C, Murphy E, et al. Regional cerebral glucose metabolism in major depressive disorder. Can J Psychiatry 1990;35(8):684–8.

[48] Kumar A, Newberg A, Alavi A, et al. Regional cerebral glucose metabolism in late-life depression and Alzheimer disease: a preliminary positron emission tomography study. Proc Natl Acad Sci U S A 1993;90(15):7019–23.

[49] Mayberg HS, Lewis PJ, Regenold W, et al. Paralimbic hypoperfusion in unipolar depression. J Nucl Med 1994;35(6):929–34.

[50] Mayberg HS, Brannan S, Mahurin R, et al. Cingulate function in depression: a potential predictor of treatment response. Neuroreport 1997;8:1057–61.

[51] Nofzinger EA, Nichols TE, Meltzer CC, et al. Changes in forebrain function from waking to REM sleep in depression: preliminary analyses of [18F]FDG PET studies. Psychiatry Res 1999;91:59–78.

[52] Bench CJ, Friston KJ, Brown RG, et al. The anatomy of melancholia—focal abnormalities of cerebral blood flow in major depression. Psychol Med 1992;22(3):607–15.

[53] Bench CJ, Friston KJ, Brown RG, et al. Regional cerebral blood flow in depression measured by positron emission tomography: the relationship with clinical dimensions. Psychol Med 1993;23(3):579–90.

[54] Dolan RJ, Bench CJ, Brown RG, et al. Regional cerebral blood flow abnormalities in depressed patients with cognitive impairment. J Neurol Neurosurg Psychiatry 1992;55(9): 768–73.

[55] Ito H, Kawashima R, Awata S, et al. Hypoperfusion in the limbic system and prefrontal cortex in depression: SPECT with anatomic standardization technique. J Nucl Med 1996;37(3):410–4.

[56] Awata S, Ito H, Konno M, et al. Regional cerebral blood flow abnormalities in late-life depression: relation to refractoriness and chronification. Psychiatry Clin Neurosci 1998;52(1):97–105.

[57] Galynker II, Cai J, Ongseng F, et al. Hypofrontality and negative symptoms in major depressive disorder. J Nucl Med 1998;39(4):608–12.

[58] Curran SM, Murray CM, Van Beck M, et al. A single photon emission computerised tomography study of regional brain function in elderly patients with major depression and with Alzheimer-type dementia. Br J Psychiatry 1993;163:155–65.

[59] Baxter LR Jr, Phelps ME, Mazziotta JC, et al. Cerebral metabolic rates for glucose in mood disorders. Studies with positron emission tomography and fluorodeoxyglucose F 18. Arch Gen Psychiatry 1985;42(5):441–7.

[60] Kuhl DE, Metter EJ, Riege WH. Patterns of cerebral glucose utilization in depression, multiple infarct dementia, and Alzheimer's disease. Res Publ Assoc Res Nerv Ment Dis 1985;63:211–26.

[61] Austin MP, Dougall N, Ross M, et al. Single photon emission tomography with 99mTc-exametazime in major depression and the pattern of brain activity underlying the psychotic/neurotic continuum. J Affect Disord 1992;26(1):31–43.

[62] Biver F, Goldman S, Delvenne V, et al. Frontal and parietal metabolic disturbances in unipolar depression. Biol Psychiatry 1994;36(6):381–8.

[63] Edmonstone Y, Austin MP, Prentice N, et al. Uptake of 99mTc-exametazime shown by single photon emission computerized tomography in obsessive-compulsive disorder compared with major depression and normal controls. Acta Psychiatr Scand 1994;90:298–303.

[64] al-Mousawi AH, Evans N, Ebmeier KP, et al. Limbic dysfunction in schizophrenia and mania. A study using 18F-labelled fluorodeoxyglucose and positron emission tomography. Br J Psychiatry 1996;169(4):509–16.

[65] Bonne O, Krausz Y, Gorfine M, et al. Cerebral hypoperfusion in medication resistant, depressed patients assessed by Tc99m HMPAO SPECT. J Affect Disord 1996;41(3):163–71.

[66] Mozley PD, Hornig-Rohan M, Woda AM, et al. Cerebral HMPAO SPECT in patients with major depression and healthy volunteers. Prog Neuropsychopharmacol Biol Psychiatry 1996;20(3):443–58.

[67] Vasile RG, Schwartz RB, Garada B, et al. Focal cerebral perfusion defects demonstrated by 99mTc-hexamethylpropyleneamine oxime SPECT in elderly depressed patients. Psychiatry Res 1996;67(1):59–70.

[68] Buchsbaum MS, Wu J, Siegel BV, et al. (1997): Effect of sertraline on regional metabolic rate in patients with affective disorder. Biol Psychiatry 1997;41(1):15–22.

[69] Hornig M, Mozley PD, Amsterdam JD. HMPAO SPECT brain imaging in treatment-resistant depression. Prog Neuropsychopharmacol Biol Psychiatry 1997;21(7):1097–114.

[70] MacHale SM, Lawrie SM, Cavanagh JT, et al. Cerebral perfusion in chronic fatigue syndrome and depression. Br J Psychiatry 2000;176:550–6.

[71] Navarro V, Gasto C, Lomena F, et al. Frontal cerebral perfusion dysfunction in elderly late-onset major depression assessed by 99MTC-HMPAO SPECT. Neuroimage 2001;14(1 Pt 1):202–5.

[72] Saxena S, Brody AL, Ho ML, et al. Cerebral metabolism in major depression and obsessive-compulsive disorder occurring separately and concurrently. Biol Psychiatry 2001;50(3): 159–70.

[73] Kimbrell TA, Ketter TA, George MS, et al. Regional cerebral glucose utilization in patients with a range of severities of unipolar depression. Biol Psychiatry 2002;51(3): 237–52.

[74] Drevets WC, Videen TO, Price JL, et al. A functional neuroanatomy study of unipolar depression. J Neurosci 1992;12:3628–41.

[75] Altshuler LL, Bartzokis G, Greider T, et al. Amygdala enlargement in bipolar disorder and hippocampal reduction in schizophrenia: an MRI study demonstrating neuroanatomic specificity. Arch Gen Psychiatry 1998;55:663–4.

[76] Altshuler LL, Bartzokis G, Greider T, et al. An MRI study of temporal lobe structures in men with bipolar disorder or schizophrenia. Biol Psychiatry 2000;48:147–62.

[77] Bremner JD, Narayan M, Anderson ER, et al. Hippocampal volume reduction in major depression. Am J Psychiatry 2000;157:115–8.

[78] Frodl T, Meisenzahl E, Zetzsche T, et al. Enlargement of the amygdale in patients with a first episode of major depression. Biol Psychiatry 2002;51:708–14.

[79] Frodl T, Meisenzahl E, Zetzsche T, et al. Larger amygdala volumes in first episode as compared to recurrent major depression and healthy control subjects. Biol Psychiatry 2003;53(4):338–44.

[80] Strakowski SM, DelBello MP, Sax KW, et al. Brain magnetic resonance imaging of structural abnormalities in bipolar disorder. Arch Gen Psychiatry 1999;56:254–60.

[81] Sheline YI, Wang PW, Gado MH, et al. Hippocampal atrophy in current major depression. Proc Natl Acad Sci U S A 1996;93:3908–13.

[82] Abercrombie HC, Schaefer SM, Larson CL, et al. Metabolic rate in the right amygdala predicts negative affect in depressed patients. Neuroreport 1998;9:3301–7.

[83] Bremner JD, Innis RB, Salomon RM, et al. Positron emission tomography measurement of cerebral metabolic correlates of tryptophan depletion-induced depressive relapse. Arch Gen Psychiatry 1997;54:364–74.

[84] Drevets WC, Price JL, Bardgett ME, et al. Glucose metabolism in the amygdala in depression: relationship to diagnostic subtype and plasma cortisol levels. Pharmacol Biochem Behav 2002;71:431–47.

[85] Ketter TA, Kimbrell TA, George MS, et al. Effects of mood and subtype on cerebral glucose metabolism in treatment-resistant bipolar disorder. Biol Psychiatry 2001;49:97–109.

[86] Ketter TA, Drevets WC. Neuroimaging studies of bipolar depression: functional neuropathology, treatment effects, and predictors of clinical response. Clin Neurosci Res 2002;2(3–4):182–92.

[87] Schneider F, Gur RE, Mozley LH, et al. Mood effects on limbic blood flow correlate with emotional self-rating: a PET study with oxygen-15 labeled water. Psychiatry Res 1995;61:265–83.

[88] Schneider F, Grodd W, Weiss U, et al. Functional MRI reveals left amygdala activation during emotion. Psychiatry Res 1997;76:75–82.

[89] Ketter TA, Wang PW. Predictors of treatment response in bipolar disorder: evidence from clinical and PET studies. J Clin Psychiatry 2002;63(Suppl 3):21–5.

[90] Fu CHY, Williams SCR, Cleare AJ, et al. Attenuation of the neural response to sad faces in major depression by antidepressant treatment: a prospective, event-related functional magnetic resonance imaging study. Arch Gen Psychiatry 2004;61:877–89.

[91] Sheline YI, Barch DM, Donnelly JM, et al. Increased amygdala response to masked emotional faces in depressed subjects resolves with antidepressant treatment: an fMRI study. Biol Psychiatry 2001;50:651–8.

[92] Yurgelun-Todd DA, Gruber SA, Kanayama G, et al. fMRI during affect discrimination in bipolar disorder. Bipolar Disord 2000;2:237–48.

[93] Siegle GJ, Steinhauer SR, Thase ME, et al. Can't shake that feeling: event-related fMRI assessment of sustained amygdala activity in response to emotional information in depressed individuals. Biol Psychiatry 2002;51:693–707.

[94] Wu JC, Gillin JC, Buchsbaum MS, et al. Effect of sleep deprivation on brain metabolism of depressed patients. Am J Psychiatry 1992;149(4):538–43.

[95] Ebert D, Feistel H, Barocka A. Effects of sleep deprivation on the limbic system and the frontal lobes in affective disorders: a study with Tc-99m-HMPAO SPECT. Psychiatry Res 1991;40(4):247–51.

[96] Drevets WC. Prefrontal cortical-amygdalar metabolism in major depression. Ann N Y Acad Sci 1999;877:614–37.

[97] Drevets WC. Neuroimaging abnormalities in the amygdala in mood disorders. Ann N Y Acad Sci 2003;985:420–44.
[98] Dougherty DD, Mayberg HS. Neuroimaging studies of treatment response: the example of major depression. In: Dougherty DD, Rauch SL, editors. Psychiatric neuroimaging research: contemporary strategies. Washington, DC: American Psychiatric Publishing; 2001. p. 179–92.
[99] Evans KC, Dougherty DD, Pollack MH, et al. Using neuroimaging to predict treatment response in mood and anxiety disorders. Ann Clin Psychiatry 2006;18: 33–42.
[100] Ebert D, Feistel H, Barocka A, et al. Increased limbic blood flow and total sleep deprivation in major depression with melancholia. Psychiatry Res 1994;55(2): 101–9.
[101] Holthoff VA, Beuthien-Baumann B, Pietrzyk U, et al. [Changes in regional cerebral perfusion in depression. SPECT monitoring of response to treatment]. Nervenarzt 1999;70(7): 620–6 [in German].
[102] Wu J, Buchsbaum MS, Gillin JC, et al. Prediction of antidepressant effects of sleep deprivation by metabolic rates in the ventral anterior cingulate and medial prefrontal cortex. Am J Psychiatry 1999;156:1149–58.
[103] Brody AL, Saxena S, Silverman DHS, et al. Brain metabolic changes in major depressive disorder from pre- to post-treatment with paroxetine. Psychiatry Res 1999;91:127–39.
[104] Pizzagalli D, Pascual-Marqui RD, Nitschke JB, et al. Anterior cingulate activity as a predictor of degree of treatment response in major depression: evidence from brain electrical tomography analysis. Am J Psychiatry 2001;158:405–15.
[105] Little JT, Ketter TA, Kimbrell TA, et al. Venlafaxine or bupropion responders but not nonresponders show baseline prefrontal and paralimbic hypometabolism compared with controls. Psychopharmacol Bull 1996;32:629–35.
[106] Canli T, Cooney RE, Goldin P, et al. Amygdala reactivity to emotional faces predicts improvement in major depression. Neuroreport 2005;16:1267–70.
[107] Dougherty DD, Weiss AP, Cosgrove GR, et al. Cerebral metabolic correlates as potential predictors of response to anterior cingulotomy for major depression. J Neurosurg 2003;99:1010–7.

The Promise of the Quantitative Electroencephalogram as a Predictor of Antidepressant Treatment Outcomes in Major Depressive Disorder

Aimee M. Hunter, PhD[a],*, Ian A. Cook, MD[b],
Andrew F. Leuchter, MD[c]

[a]Laboratory of Brain, Behavior, and Pharmacology, Semel Institute for Neuroscience
and Human Behavior at UCLA, Department of Psychiatry and Biobehavioral Sciences,
David Geffen School of Medicine at UCLA, 760 Westwood Plaza Rm. 37-359,
Los Angeles, CA 90024-1759, USA
[b]Laboratory of Brain, Behavior, and Pharmacology, Semel Institute for Neuroscience
and Human Behavior at UCLA, Department of Psychiatry and Biobehavioral Sciences,
David Geffen School of Medicine at UCLA, 760 Westwood Plaza Rm. 37-351,
Los Angeles, CA 90024-1759, USA
[c]Laboratory of Brain, Behavior, and Pharmacology, Semel Institute for Neuroscience
and Human Behavior at UCLA, Department of Psychiatry and Biobehavioral Sciences,
David Geffen School of Medicine at UCLA, 760 Westwood Plaza Rm. 37-452,
Los Angeles, CA 90024-1759, USA

WHY DO WE NEED PREDICTORS OF ANTIDEPRESSANT TREATMENT OUTCOME?

A large percentage of patients (30%–53%) fail to respond to an initial course of antidepressant medication [1–3], and for those who do respond clinical improvement often takes a long time. Results of the recently completed multisite study of Sequenced Treatment Alternatives to Relieve Depression, reviewed extensively by Nierenberg and Fava in this issue, highlight this point. With 2876 analyzable participants, this landmark study is the single largest trial of treatment outcomes for depression to date; in contrast to many clinical trials, minimal exclusionary criteria ensured that participants were representative of real-world, treatment-seeking outpatients who had nonpsychotic major depressive disorder. At study outset, all subjects were treated with the maximum tolerated dose of citalopram (up to 60 mg) for up to 14 weeks. Even with aggressive dosing, this representative selective serotonin reuptake

This work was supported by grant R01-MH069217 and contract N01 MH90003/GMO-010111 from the National Institute of Mental Health (IAC), grant R01 AT 002479 from the National Center for Complementary and Alternative Medicine (AFL), and a grant from Aspect Medical Systems (IAC).

*Corresponding author. E-mail address: amhunter@ucla.edu (A.M. Hunter).

0193-953X/07/$ – see front matter
doi:10.1016/j.psc.2006.12.002

inhibitor (SSRI) showed only modest effectiveness. Examining a response criterion of a reduction of 50% or more on the 16-item Quick Inventory of Depressive Symptomatology, Self-Report (QIDS-SR) and a remission criterion of five or lower on the QIDS-SR, only 47% of subjects responded and 29% remitted. Moreover, even for subjects who responded and/or remitted after 14 weeks of treatment, symptomatic improvement was slow. After 6 weeks, only about two thirds (65.2%) of ultimate responders had responded, and just over half (52.9%) of ultimate remitters had remitted [3]. These data mirror the typical experience in clinical practice; that is, response or remission to a given medication is uncertain, and it takes a long time to determine outcome.

The inability to predict a patient's response to a particular treatment can lead to a delay in effective treatment, which in turn can have a number of deleterious consequences. Without any reliable means of predicting outcome, patients and physicians are left to use a trial-and-error strategy in which the trial often lasts 6 to 12 weeks. Patients who do not respond to an initial treatment must endure subsequent trials to determine the effectiveness of different regimens, and many abandon treatment while still symptomatic [4]. The most apparent consequence of delayed effective treatment is that patients continue to suffer from the symptoms of depression including increased risk for suicide [5]. There also is evidence that prolonged depression is associated with deleterious effects on the central nervous system. Major depression has been associated with reduced hippocampal volume [6], and longer durations of untreated depressive episodes have been associated with lower hippocampal volume [7]. Patients who do not respond to their first antidepressant trial are at increased risk for never receiving adequate treatment [4], and delays in effective treatment are associated with a poorer prognosis for the course of illness over subsequent episodes. A longer index episode (>12 weeks) has been associated with a 37% lower rate of recovery in subsequent episodes [8]. One study examining the impact of 16 sociodemographic and clinical factors identified rapid remission as the most important predictor of favorable long-term outcome [9]. In addition to health concerns, medical expenditures also increase with increasing numbers of ineffective treatment trials. A study of 7737 depressed subjects found higher inpatient, outpatient, and pharmaceutical health care costs with increasing numbers of changes in antidepressant treatment regimen [10]. The introduction of reliable predictors of response to treatment thus could potentially shorten the course of treatment and improve long-term treatment outcomes in depression.

CLINICAL AND PHYSIOLOGIC PREDICTORS OF ANTIDEPRESSANT RESPONSE

The clinical relevance of predicting response has driven a great deal of exploration of possible sociodemographic, clinical, and pretreatment physiologic predictors [11–16]. Many inconsistencies exist across studies, however, and most factors that seem to have heuristic value in differentiating groups of responders or nonresponders have not proven to be reliable pretreatment predictors of response for individual patients [17–21]. As yet, none has proven sufficiently useful to be adopted into clinical practice for predicting treatment response [14–22]. A few notable measurements have begun to demonstrate increased levels of reliability and accuracy as predictors of antidepressant response. For example, considerable data in the burgeoning literature on pharmacogenetics have linked response to SSRI treatment with genetic variants in the sequences coding for specific molecules including the serotonin (5-HT) transporter, 5-HT-2A-receptor, tryptophan hydroxylase, brain-derived neurotrophic factor, G protein beta3 subunit, interleukin-1beta, and angiotensin-converting enzyme, but with inconsistencies among results [23]. Further work with large patient samples stratified for intervening variables is needed before drawing more definite conclusions [24]. Although there is hope is that the identification of key genetic components eventually will facilitate individualized treatment planning (so-called "personalized medicine"), small variances of analyzed polymorphisms may diminish optimism for immediate application at the clinical level [25]. In a line of work examining functional brain asymmetry, perceptual asymmetry as assessed using dichotic listening tests has been demonstrated repeatedly as a predictor of response to fluoxetine with some evidence of clinically meaningful accuracy; however, gender-dependent relationships between predictor and outcome variables require further study [26–28]. Also, it is unknown whether this marker is medication specific.

Other investigations have examined changes in physiologic function during antidepressant treatment as biomarkers of therapeutic response. Several studies using positron emission tomography (PET) to assess cerebral metabolism during treatment have reported differences in prefrontal and/or cingulate activity between responders and nonresponders to antidepressant medications. Most studies report that metabolism increases in ventral paralimbic areas or in the caudate nucleus during effective antidepressant treatment [29]; cortical metabolism, however, has been reported either to increase or decrease, depending upon the study [30,31]. Most studies of cerebral blood flow, as well as most recent studies of cerebral metabolism, indicate that a decrease in cerebral perfusion in dorsolateral prefrontal cortex is associated with effective antidepressant treatment. In reports of a relatively large sample of subjects who had depression, investigators found decreases in perfusion in prefrontal cortex [32,33]. Previous findings also have reported decreases in prefrontal cerebral perfusion in subjects responding to various antidepressant medications [34]. Other investigators have reported decreases in prefrontal cortex metabolism in subjects responding to paroxetine treatment [35,36]. Despite these encouraging findings, the real-world clinical application of PET scans for predicting treatment outcomes may be limited. Dosimetry concerns impose limitations on the safe use of radioactive tracers for serial scanning. This technology also is costly and invasive, and access is limited outside a research setting.

ELECTROENCEPHALOGRAPHIC PREDICTORS OF ANTIDEPRESSANT OUTCOMES

Overview

Electroencephalography (EEG) has long held appeal as an easily accessible technique to measure central nervous system activity. Since Hans Berger's first recording of the human EEG in the mid-1920s and early demonstrations that drugs that influence human behavior also produce obvious effects on human EEG, numerous attempts have been made to apply the recording of electrical activity from scalp electrodes to a wide range of psychiatric concerns including diagnosis, treatment selection, and drug development. Historically, the field has covered a broad range of applications and methodologies. Researchers have examined various spontaneous and activation-induced EEG features measured at different time-points, recorded using a variety of electrode montages, and analyzed using different approaches. Moreover, few early studies controlled for potentially confounding variables. Although the lack of standardization makes comparisons among early findings difficult, and the absence of controls leaves open the interpretation of results, these early reports provide the first evidence of the potential capability of quantitative electroencephalography (QEEG) measurements to predict clinical outcome to antidepressant medications. More recently, studies have begun to refine methods to give EEG markers greater predictive capability and to standardize those methods to allow replication of results. In addition, some newer studies have used more rigorous experimental designs and controls, thus allowing greater certainty in interpretations of the observed relationships between EEG markers and clinical response during treatment with antidepressant medication.

Rationale Behind Electroencephalographic Markers of Response

A potential EEG predictor of antidepressant response can be measured (1) before treatment (ie, as a baseline or pretreatment measure), (2) shortly after start of drug, or (3) as a "change variable" or "change indicator" describing change in the EEG from a pretreatment baseline to a time-point after initiating treatment. In any case, to have clinical utility as a predictor, the EEG measure of course must precede the clinical response. The assumption underlying a baseline EEG indicator is that state and/or trait factors reflected in the EEG are related to how the subject will respond to antidepressant medication. The assumptions behind an EEG predictor measured sometime early after the onset of drug treatment are that (1) antidepressant medication produces changes in the EEG soon after beginning treatment, and (2) identifiable medication-related EEG changes are reliably linked to later clinical changes. A subject's brain state or change in brain state after a brief period of antidepressant treatment presumably reflects the interaction between patient factors and exposure to medication and would be a leading indicator of eventual clinical trajectory.

Early Work Suggesting Relationships Among Electroencephalographic Findings, Symptoms of Depression, and Antidepressant Medication Effects

A considerable body of research supports the assertion that antidepressant medication effects are physiologically detectable in the EEG. Prior work in the "pharmaco-EEG" tradition has shown that administration of antidepressant compounds to healthy subjects produces reliable EEG changes within hours of dosing [37–47]. Although there are reproducible EEG effects of antidepressant medications across subjects, variances in the EEG response also have been noted [48]. Differences in medication effects on the EEG have been linked to individual differences in the pre-exposure EEG [48], suggesting that the baseline EEG may indeed capture state or trait aspects of central nervous system function that moderate subsequent effects of medication on the central nervous system.

Use of the EEG to predict antidepressant outcome has roots in an early study that examined pretreatment EEG and the change from pre- to post-treatment EEG as potential predictors of outcome to amitriptyline and pirlindole [49]. Responder versus nonresponder groups assessed after 4 weeks of treatment were differentiated on the basis of both their pretreatment baseline EEGs and pre- to posttreatment EEG changes after 4 weeks. Responder groups were distinguished by a number of EEG parameters, especially in the alpha range. Among other features, responders were characterized by left lateralization of baseline alpha power, decreases in absolute alpha power, and increases in slower frequencies over 4 weeks. Although EEGs were recorded from occipital, central, and frontal regions, only occipital regions were evaluated in the primary report. Later reanalyses of these data examined the topographical distribution of alpha activity across recording regions and found lateralized differences in anterior as well as posterior regions between responders and nonresponders [50,51]. Some EEG correlates of response were medication specific [50,51], whereas others were observed with both medications [49].

A later study examining EEG predictors of 3-week response to the heterocyclic antidepressants clomipramine and maprotiline found that early changes in the EEG (ie, changes from baseline to 2 hours after the first daily drug infusion) distinguished between later responders and nonresponders to either medication [52]. In that study, the EEG measure used as a predictor measure was the frequency of non-A epochs (ie, 2-second epochs that do not represent alpha activity) as calculated using a novel procedure to quantify spatiotemporal changes in alpha activity [53].

Lateralized baseline alpha power was associated with response to fluoxetine in a study of 53 depressed adults [27]. Left dominant pretreatment values of alpha power (indicative of greater right hemisphere activation) were associated with 12-week response as measured using the Clinical Global Impression Improvement scale. This predictive relationship was evident for women but not for men.

Pretreatment baseline and postdrug change differences in theta-band log transformed relative power were found to distinguish responders from nonresponders to 4 weeks of open-label treatment with the tricyclic antidepressant imipramine [54]. At pretreatment, responders exhibited significantly less overall theta power; pretreatment differences in other frequencies were not significant. Acute (3 hours after initial dose) postdrug change in overall theta power distinguished responders from nonresponders. Considering EEG changes over the first 2 weeks of treatment, responders showed significantly greater increments in anterior theta power than did nonresponders.

In a study examining baseline EEG predictors of response to the SSRI agent paroxetine, lower baseline relative theta power again was associated with greater improvement [55]. Of note, all significant pretreatment indicators were localized to frontal brain regions. This finding is in contrast to the study of imipramine that reported a positive association between overall lower baseline theta power and response [54]. Differences in these findings could be related to different mechanisms of action between tricyclic and SSRI medications.

Taken together, these reports provide evidence suggesting that pre- and posttreatment EEG measurements (especially measurements in alpha and theta bands and potentially lateralized and frontal measurements) are related to later clinical outcome of antidepressant treatment. These reports show subtle but statistically significant EEG differences between groups of responders and nonresponders; however, the considerable overlap in the distribution of values for responders and nonresponders limits the predictive validity for individual patients. Another consideration regarding these studies is that none examined placebo-control conditions; therefore, a limit of these investigations is that it is not possible to discern whether the EEG findings were related generally to clinical improvement or more specifically to drug efficacy (specific versus nonspecific or placebolike effects).

Quantitative Electroencephalographic Biomarkers: a New Wave of Accuracy in Predicting Antidepressant Response

Neurobiologic conceptual model underlying relationships between frontal theta measurements (relative power and cordance) and antidepressant response

Several lines of reasoning support the rationale for examining frontal EEG measurements in the theta band (4–8 Hz) in relation to antidepressant medication effects and changes in depressive symptoms. The underlying neurobiologic conceptual model draws on prior work indicating that (1) activity in anterior cingulate and dorsolateral prefrontal regions is related both to depression and changes in mood in response to treatment; (2) prefrontal theta activity is associated with other measurements of cortical activity in the anterior cingulate and seems to be related to network processing of affective information; and (3) the effects of antidepressant medication produce alterations in theta band activity.

A consistent finding in neuroimaging studies from independent research groups is that of abnormal metabolism or perfusion in the dorsolateral prefrontal cortex and/or the anterior cingulate cortex in depressed subjects [29,30,36,56–62]. Prefrontal and cingulate regions also figure consistently and prominently in studies using EEG to examine brain function associated with depressed mood [27,63–69], and these regions also have been examined using functional MRI [70,71]. Networks of projecting white-matter fibers connect these regions, both neuroanatomically and functionally [72–76]. The importance of these anatomic tracts in this context is that rhythmic theta activity recorded at the scalp in prefrontal channels may reflect both the intrinsic activity originating in the dorsolateral prefrontal cortex and the projected rhythms that are generated in deep locations (eg, the anterior cingulate) and influence activity in the cortex nearer to the recording electrodes.

Theta band activity in particular has been examined with regard to coordinated activity between the midline prefrontal and cingulate regions. Studies that combined surface EEG recordings and magnetoencephalographic (MEG) data have indicated that surface theta rhythms recorded from prefrontal channels are correlated with deep theta MEG activity in the anterior cingulate [77,78]. Activity in the theta band seems to be important to the integration of activity across distributed neural networks [79,80]. Shifts in theta band activity also have been particularly linked with processing emotionally related stimuli and meditation-related changes in emotional state [81–84].

Antidepressant compounds [54,55,85–88] and treatment with electroconvulsive therapy [89] have been shown to alter theta activity. Pretreatment theta cordance measured from electrodes overlying the cingulate cortex has been related to the response to electroconvulsive therapy in major depressive disorder (MDD) [90]. Using EEG tomography, pretreatment theta activity associated with antidepressant response has been localized to the anterior cingulate [63].

Theta band relative power
Several naturalistic studies using open-label, flexible-dose SSRI treatment have demonstrated the predictive capability of theta band relative power measured from frontal electrodes. In a cohort of 36 adult outpatients meeting criteria for MDD, frontal theta band relative power 1 week after start of drug was significantly lower in responders than in nonresponders [91]. Response was defined as a reduction of 50% or more in scores on the 17-item Hamilton Depression Rating Scale ($HamD_{17}$) from baseline to week eight. Lower theta band relative power at 1 week also correlated with percent improvement in the $HamD_{17}$ score over 8 weeks. Importantly, this measure predicted response with 83% overall accuracy (76% sensitivity, 93% specificity) and .88 area under the receiver operating curve. This essential finding was replicated by the same group of investigators in a larger sample of 68 patients who had MDD treated with SSRIs [92]. Again, frontal theta band relative power 1 week after start of drug was significantly lower in responders than in nonresponders and was negatively correlated with the magnitude of clinical improvement. The predictor yielded an overall accuracy of 67% with 71% sensitivity and 61% specificity.

Another analysis of frontal theta band relative power, also from the same investigators, examined 52 subjects who had MDD grouped by depressive subtype (melancholic, atypical, or typical) [93] and treated naturalistically. Baseline frontal theta band relative power was significantly lower in SSRI responders than in nonresponders, and the difference in frontal theta band relative power between responders and nonresponders was similar across clinical subtypes. Baseline theta band relative power alone predicted response with 71% accuracy (72% sensitivity, 70% specificity) and in combination with measurements of theta band relative power at 1 week resulted in improved prediction (79% accuracy, 84% sensitivity, and 70% specificity.) Here, the addition of the week one measure added to the ability to correctly identify responders.

An independent study of 22 outpatients who had MDD examined frontal theta band relative power measurements as predictors of 8-week response to citalopram [94]. Mean decreases in frontal theta band relative power were observed in responders but not in nonresponders at weeks one, two, and four. The decrease in theta band relative power 2 weeks after start of medication was significantly greater in treatment responders than in nonresponders, and decreases predicted response with 73% accuracy (73% sensitivity, 73% specificity).

These studies are comparable in many respects. Each used identical, automated EEG recording methods to measure frontal theta band relative power, examined outpatients who had MDD receiving open-label treatment with SSRIs, and assessed response/nonresponse outcome as an improvement of 50% or more on the HamD$_{17}$ scale after 8 weeks of treatment. Each of these studies demonstrated significant associations between clinical response to antidepressant medication and lower frontal theta band activity or decreases in frontal theta band activity within the first 2 weeks after start of medication. Strong predictive capability was demonstrated for frontal theta band relative power biomarkers, but there was some variability in the EEG time-points used as predictors in these studies of theta band relative power. Predictive capability was shown either for baseline, week one, or change at week two EEG measurements, depending on the study; therefore they cannot be viewed as direct replications of the same finding. Furthermore, because these studies did not examine control subjects treated with placebo, the capacity of these indicators to discriminate between specific response to medication and nonspecific effects is unknown.

Quantitative electroencephalographic cordance development
Cordance is a measure that combines absolute and relative power with the goal of extracting information with greater physiologic meaning from QEEG. Absolute power, the amount of power in a frequency band at a given electrode (measured in μV^2), and relative power, the percentage of power contained in a frequency band relative to the total power across the entire spectrum, are associated inconsistently with direct measurements of cerebral

energy use, making their physiologic significance unclear [95]. For example, relationships between EEG power measurements and perfusion or metabolism show considerable variability across frequency bands and sites [96,97], with some studies showing only weak associations [98]. Absolute power and relative power are, in fact, complementary measurements of brain activity [99] that have independent associations with perfusion [100]. Cordance combines traditional absolute power and relative power measurements to achieve a stronger association with cerebral perfusion than is seen with either measure alone. A detailed description of how cordance is calculated is provided elsewhere [101].

Several studies have demonstrated relationships between QEEG cordance and other physiologic measurements. In a series of outpatient case studies, cordance was reported to have strong associations with other measurements of brain structure and function including white-matter lesions detected on MRI, metabolism measured by PET using fluorodeoxyglucose, and perfusion measured by hexamethylpropyleneamine oxime single-photon emission computed tomography (SPECT) [95]. A larger study examining 27 outpatients who had degenerative or vascular dementia showed that cordance had a stronger association with perfusion (measured using SPECT) than either absolute or relative power measurements alone, and this relationship held across multiple brain regions as evidenced by data from frontal, temporal, and occipital electrode sites [102]. Finally, a study of normal healthy subjects compared associations between perfusion (measured using O^{15} PET) and QEEG measurements including absolute power, relative power, and cordance [101]. Of the three EEG measurements examined, cordance was found to have a moderately strong association with perfusion and was the strongest of the measurements examined, both during a resting state and motor task performance. In addition, cordance was as effective as PET in detecting lateralized activation associated with a motor task; EEG power measurements did not detect this activation.

Theta cordance as a predictor of antidepressant treatment outcomes. The first systematic report to indicate that theta cordance might be sensitive to pharmacotherapy interventions was made in the context of a study that used cordance to assess cerebral energy use in late-life depression [100]. QEEG theta cordance measurements were obtained for 27 depressed subjects and 27 matched controls with the hypothesis that depressed subjects would show overall alterations consistent with the decreases in perfusion and metabolism seen using PET [59] or SPECT [103]. Results supported the hypothesis and demonstrated differences in global and regional cordance between depressed and control subjects. It is important for response prediction that cordance patterns were found to differ significantly between depressed subjects who were being treated with antidepressant medication and those who were not. This observation, albeit cross-sectional, suggested that theta cordance might be sensitive to changes in brain function attributable to antidepressant treatment.

The relationship between theta cordance and treatment response was explored in a series of individual cases that illustrated frontal decreases in theta cordance as early as 48 hours after beginning medication preceding clinical improvement in depressed outpatients receiving open-label treatment with SSRI or serotonin-norepinephrine reuptake inhibitor (SNRI) medications [31]. Later, a larger case series prospectively examined decreases in prefrontal cordance as a predictor of 2-month outcome in seven subjects who had major depression receiving naturalistic open-label treatment with SSRI or SNRI antidepressants [104]. Subjects were free of psychotropic medications for 2 weeks before enrollment in the study. All four responders showed large decreases in cordance 48 hours and 1 week after initiating medication. None of the three nonresponders showed this pattern; one showed only a slight decrease, and the other two nonresponders showed frank increases in prefrontal theta band cordance. Using a simple dichotomous decrease/no decrease predictor (in which decrease predicted response), change in prefrontal theta band cordance yielded an overall accuracy of 86%, with 100% sensitivity and 67% specificity.

Data from individual cases prompted the first hypothesis-driven placebo-controlled study of theta band cordance as a potential biomarker of antidepressant response [105]. Decreases in prefrontal theta band cordance at 48 hours and at 1 week after start of medication were hypothesized to predict 8-week antidepressant response (final $HamD_{17} \leq 10$). Data were pooled from 51 depressed patients across two placebo-controlled studies that used fluoxetine or venlafaxine, respectively, as the active medication. There was a trend finding at 48 hours, and at 1week change in prefrontal theta band cordance significantly distinguished medication responders from all other groups (medication nonresponders, placebo responders, and placebo nonresponders). In addition, the degree of change in prefrontal cordance was significantly associated with degree of response. Using prefrontal cordance decrease/no decrease as a dichotomous predictor of response accurately classified 9 of 13 medication responders (69%) and 9 or 12 medication nonresponders (75%) for an overall accuracy of 72%. Decreases in prefrontal theta band cordance did not predict response among subjects assigned randomly to placebo. In fact, a separate study of the same 51 subjects revealed a distinctly different pattern of change (4- and 8-week increases in prefrontal cordance) for placebo responders as compared with all other groups [106].

The finding of early decrease in prefrontal cordance as a predictor of response has been replicated by the same group of investigators and by an independent research team. In a study of patients who had treatment-resistant depression, prefrontal theta band cordance EEG measurements were obtained a cohort of 12 outpatients at baseline and approximately 1 week after beginning a new treatment [107]. These patients had not responded to monotherapy and were beginning a new treatment as prescribed by their treating psychiatrists. In contrast to earlier studies that had used a drug-free interval or drug washout period before obtaining the baseline EEG [104,105], these treatment-resistant subjects were evaluated without a drug-free interval between trials. Response was evaluated after 8 to 10 weeks. Of six responders, five showed an early decrease in cordance; only two of the six nonresponders showed an early cordance decrease. The predictor yielded accurate classification for 75% of the subjects. Findings using cordance have been replicated independently in a study of 17 depressed inpatients receiving open-label treatment with antidepressants from a variety of classifications [108]. Prefrontal theta band cordance decreases after 1 week predicted response (>50% reduction of Montgomery-Asberg Depression Rating Scale scores after 4 weeks of treatment) with an overall accuracy of 88% (100% sensitivity, 83% specificity). In a pooled analysis of 54 subjects from three studies across investigative teams, decreases in prefrontal cordance yielded an overall accuracy of 78% [109].

Across studies of MDD subjects treated with various antidepressant medications, decreases in prefrontal theta band cordance 1 week after start of medication have predicted response consistently with overall accuracy ranging from 72% to 88%. Examination of this predictor in randomized, double-blind, placebo-controlled trials has demonstrated specificity for this marker as an indicator of medication efficacy.

Future Directions Using Spontaneous Electroencephalographic Measurements to Predict Other Antidepressant Outcomes

Recent evidence suggests that EEG measurements might be useful in predicting other positive outcomes as well as negative outcomes of antidepressant treatment (ie, treatment-emergent adverse events. Although most studies to date examining QEEG predictors of clinical outcome have focused on treatment response (typically $\geq 50\%$ improvement in symptoms or a final $HamD_{17}$ score ≤ 10), there is growing emphasis on remission (eg, final Ham-D score ≤ 7 or ≤ 5) as the endpoint goal of treatment. Although prefrontal channels seem to predict response with a high degree of accuracy, recent evidence suggests that electrodes overlying the midline and right frontal region may predict remission [110,111]. With regard to treatment-emergent adverse events, a promising new line of work suggests that EEG markers also may be able to predict worsening of somatic and mood symptoms. EEG markers have been linked to the overall occurrence of common side effects including headache, nausea, and sexual dysfunction [112] and to the emergence of increased thoughts of suicide [92] reported during antidepressant treatment.

OTHER ELECTROENCEPHALOGRAPHIC-RELATED PREDICTORS OF ANTIDEPRESSANT OUTCOMES

Loudness Dependence of Auditory Evoked Potentials

In addition to measurements of spontaneous EEG activity, such as relative power and cordance, measurements of brain response to a stimulus have been examined as predictors of treatment response. A variety of preclinical and clinical studies have suggested that the loudness dependence of auditory evoked potentials (LDAEP) may reflect activity in the brain's serotonergic system. These auditory evoked potentials arise from activity in the primary auditory cortex and can be studied using dipole source analysis [113]; the ratio of N1/P2 amplitude values increases with increasing tone loudness during auditory stimulation, and LDAEP values are inversely related to central serotonergic activity. Patients who had a strong LDAEP (a marker of a low serotonergic state) before treatment responded significantly better to SSRI medications than did patients who had a lower LDAEP (and, presumably, high or normal serotonergic activity) [114–119]. One study has examined the predictive value of the LDAEP in relation to treatment with the SNRI reboxetine. In contrast to the direction of amplitude changes associated with SSRI response, lower pretreatment intensity-dependent N1 amplitude slopes were significantly associated with reboxetine response, suggesting that LDAEP differentially predicts clinical response to serotonergic versus noradrenergic antidepressant psychopharmacotherapy [120]. As with the approaches described previously in this article, the LDAEP method shows promise in differentiating between patients who may or may not respond to a particular medication; further independent replication under controlled conditions will help clarify how it might best be used for guiding treatment decisions in clinical care.

Nonlinear Measurements of Brain Physiology

EEG power and cordance are both linear measurements of the EEG power spectrum. A nonlinear measure of EEG activity, the bispectrum, also has been examined for use in detecting pretreatment differences between responders and nonresponders to antidepressant treatment. The bispectrum quantifies phase and power coupling between EEG components [121] and could offer a complementary measurement of regional brain activity. In an investigation of adult outpatients treated with fluoxetine, venlafaxine, or placebo [122], bispectrum values were calculated for frequency triples of the form [f1, f2, f1+f2] at 1 Hz resolution using a single frontotemporal channel (T3-Fp1). Across all treatment groups, the bispectrum in the range [12 Hz < f1 < 24 Hz, f2 < 6 Hz] was higher in the more severely depressed patients, with a significant correlation between $HamD_{17}$ score and bispectrum value. Additionally, there were baseline differences between responders and nonresponders to medication. Further replications and extensions of that work are underway, and bispectrum-based measurements might be combined with cordance or other linear measurements to create a composite biomarker with improved predictive accuracy.

HOW MIGHT INFORMATION FROM ELECTROENCEPHALOGRAPHIC PREDICTORS BE USED IN CLINICAL PRACTICE?

Reliable prediction of antidepressant treatment outcomes would have benefit regardless of whether indicators for a given antidepressant regimen point toward response or failure for a patient. Pretreatment, as compared with postdrug, indicators might be interpreted slightly differently. The value of a positive EEG change indicator would be to provide the patient and physician with some degree of assurance that continued treatment will be fruitful and to avoid unnecessary (and perhaps ineffective) switching and/or augmentation of medications. Increased confidence in a positive outcome also could encourage treatment adherence even as patients contend with side effects that can peak before therapeutic effects are realized. In the case of a negative change indicator, the probably ineffective treatment regimen could be changed far sooner than is current common practice, and the new regimen could be initiated shortly thereafter. Evidence from a study of subjects who had stage I treatment-resistant depression suggests that the predictive capability of QEEG cordance biomarkers does not require a drug-free interval between treatments [107]. Positive baseline indicators could suggest that a given individual is generally suitable for antidepressant medication whether because of state or trait factors; pretreatment EEG biomarkers (LDAEPs notwithstanding) have not been studied extensively with respect to their ability to predict differential response to different medications. The value of a negative baseline indicator for antidepressant response is unknown, although it is possible that other types of interventions would be more effective for individuals who have a poor prognostic indicator for pharmacotherapy. Another interpretation is that a negative baseline indicator suggests that the transient state of the individual is not conducive to antidepressant response at that time. In this view, medication-free measurements repeated over time might change from an unfavorable to a favorable indicator for pharmacotherapy, thus identifying a particular time during which initiation of antidepressant treatment would likely lead to clinical response or remission.

CAVEATS AND CAUTIONS

The comparatively low cost, high patient acceptability, and technological ease of performing QEEG data collection and analysis can be viewed as strengths of this approach. On the other hand, these same attributes mean that there is a low barrier to entry in the field, and individuals and groups with little training or experience can gather QEEG data on patients or research subjects. The reliability and interpretability of these data may be inconsistent or worse.

The conclusions that can be drawn from any innovative clinical research study need to be subjected to scientific scrutiny through peer review and independent replication of findings before they can be considered for use in advancing clinical care, whether the innovation is a new molecule designed for therapeutic use or a technology proposed for guiding treatment. Unfortunately, the low barriers to entry in the QEEG arena have meant that naively designed, poorly executed, or inappropriately analyzed data are not subjected consistently to the normal checks and balances of the scientific method, and systems purporting to diagnose and/or provide guidance for care are available without having been subjected to rigorous review expected of other advances in biomedical research. The research and clinical communities therefore must be attuned to the reality that not all "QEEG" systems represent the same measure or technique. Only through thoughtful consideration of each method separately can the claims advanced for a particular technique be assessed. After this type of careful review, methods for which there is an adequate evidence base enter the mainstream of care.

SUMMARY

Recent studies have shown overall accuracy rates of 72% to 88% using baseline and/or 1-week change in QEEG biomarkers to predict clinical outcome to treatment with various antidepressant medications. In some cases, findings have been replicated across academic institutions and have been studied in the context of randomized, placebo-controlled trials. Recent EEG findings are corroborated by studies that use techniques with greater spatial resolution (eg, PET, MEG) in localizing brain regions pertinent to clinical response. As such, EEG measurements increasingly are validated by other physiologic measurements that have the ability to assess deeper brain structures. Continued progress along these lines may lead to the realized promise of QEEG biomarkers as predictors of antidepressant treatment outcome in routine clinical practice. In the larger context, use of QEEG technology to predict antidepressant response in major depression may mean that more patients will achieve response and remission with less of the trial-and-error approach that currently accompanies antidepressant treatment.

Acknowledgments

The authors thank Jennifer Pacheco and Elaine Stautzenberger for assistance in preparing the manuscript.

References

[1] Baldessarini RJ. Current status of antidepressants: clinical pharmacology and therapy. J Clin Psychiatry 1989;50:117–26.
[2] Rush AJ, Carmody TJ, Donahue RM, et al. Response in relation to baseline anxiety levels in major depressive disorder treated with bupropion sustained release or sertraline. Neuropsychopharmacology 2001;25:131–8.
[3] Trivedi M, Rush A, Wisniewski S, et al. Evaluation of outcomes with citalopram for depression using measurement-based care in STAR*D: implications for clinical practice. Am J Psychiatry 2006;163(1):28–40.
[4] Katzelnick DJ, Kobak K, Greist JK, et al. Predictors of adequate dose and duration of antidepressant medication for depression in a HMO. Poster 86 presented at the 37th annual meeting of the New Clinical Drug Evaluation Unit (NCDEU). Boca Raton, May 27–30, 1997.
[5] Simon GE, Savarino J, Operskalski B, et al. Suicide risk during antidepressant treatment. Am J Psychiatry 2006;163(1):41–7.
[6] Bremner J, Narayan M, Anderson E, et al. Hippocampal volume reduction in major depression. Am J Psychiatry 2000;157(1):115–8.
[7] Sheline Y, Gado M, Kraemer H. Untreated depression and hippocampal volume loss. Am J Psychiatry 2003;160(8):1516–8.
[8] Spijker J, de Graaf R, Bijl R, et al. Determinants of persistence of major depressive episodes in the general population. Results from the Netherlands Mental Health Survey and Incidence Study (NEMESIS). J Affect Disord 2004;81(3):231–40.

[9] Szadoczky E, Rozsa S, Zambori J, et al. Predictors for 2-year outcome of major depressive episode. J Affect Disord 2004;83(1):49–57.

[10] Russell J, Hawkins K, Ozminkowski R, et al. The cost consequences of treatment-resistant depression. J Clin Psychiatry 2004;65(3):341–7.

[11] Bielski RJ, Friedel RO. Prediction of tricyclic antidepressant response: a critical review. Arch Gen Psychiatry 1976;33(12):1479–89.

[12] Ananth J. Clinical prediction of antidepressant response. Int Pharmacopsychiatry 1978;13(2):69–93.

[13] Balon R. Biological predictors of antidepressant treatment outcome. Clin Neuropharmacol 1989;12(3):195–214.

[14] Joyce PR, Paykel ES. Predictors of drug response in depression. Arch Gen Psychiatry 1989;46(1):89–99.

[15] Kocsis JH. New issues in the prediction of antidepressant response. Psychopharmacol Bull 1990;26(1):49–53.

[16] Goodwin FK. Predictors of antidepressant response. Bull Menninger Clin 1993;57(2): 146–60.

[17] Mulder RT, Joyce PR, Sullivan PF, et al. Intimate bonds in depression. J Affect Disord 1996;40:175–8.

[18] Small GW, Hamilton SH, Bystritsky A, et al. Clinical response predictors in a double-blind, placebo-controlled trial of fluoxetine for geriatric major depression. Fluoxetine Collaborative Study Group. Int Psychogeriatr 1995;7(Suppl):41–53.

[19] Cohn JB, Wilcox C. A comparison of fluoxetine, imipramine, and placebo in patients with major depressive disorder. J Clin Psychiatry 1985;46:26–31.

[20] Nierenberg AA, McLean NE, Alpert JE, et al. Early nonresponse to fluoxetine as a predictor of poor 8-week outcome. Am J Psychiatry 1995;152:1500–3.

[21] Nierenberg AA. Predictors of response to antidepressants general principles and clinical implications. Psychiatr Clin North Am 2003;26(2):345–52.

[22] Schmauss M, Erfurth A. Predicting antidepressive treatment success–critical review and perspectives. Fortschr Neurol Psychiatr 1993;61:274–83.

[23] Serretti A, Artioli P. The pharmacogenomics of selective serotonin reuptake inhibitors. Pharmacogenomics J 2004;4(4):233–44.

[24] Lerer B, Macciardi F. Pharmacogenetics of antidepressant and mood-stabilizing drugs: a review of candidate-gene studies and future research directions. Int J Neuropsychopharmacol 2002;5(3):255–75.

[25] Serretti A, Artioli P, Quartesan R. Pharmacogenetics in the treatment of depression: pharmacodynamic studies. Pharmacogenet Genomics 2005;15(2): 61–7.

[26] Bruder GE, Otto MW, McGrath PJ, et al. Dichotic listening before and after fluoxetine treatment for major depression: relations of laterality to therapeutic response. Neuropsychopharmacology 1996;15(2):171–9.

[27] Bruder GE, Stewart JW, Tenke CE, et al. Electroencephalographic and perceptual asymmetry differences between responders and nonresponders to an SSRI antidepressant. Biol Psychiatry 2001;49(5):416–25.

[28] Bruder GE, Stewart JW, McGrath PJ, et al. Dichotic listening tests of functional brain asymmetry predict response to fluoxetine in depressed women and men. Neuropsychopharmacology 2004;29(9):1752–61.

[29] Mayberg HS, Brannan SK, Mahurin RK, et al. Cingulate function in depression: a potential predictor of treatment response. Neuroreport 1997;8:1057–61.

[30] Kennedy SH, Evans KR, Kruger S, et al. Changes in regional brain glucose metabolism measured with positron emission tomography after paroxetine treatment of major depression. Am J Psychiatry 2001;158(6):899–905.

[31] Leuchter A, Cook I, Uijtdehaage S, et al. Brain structure and function and the outcomes of treatment for depression. J Clin Psychiatry 1997;58(Suppl 16):22–31.

[32] Drevets WC, Raichle ME. Neuroanatomical circuits in depression: implications for treatment mechanisms. 30th Annual Meeting of the American College of Neuropsychopharmacology (1991, San Juan, Puerto Rico). Psychopharmacol Bull 1992;28:261–74.
[33] Drevets WC. Geriatric depression: brain imaging correlates and pharmacologic considerations. J Clin Psychiatry 1994;55(Suppl A):71–82, 98–100.
[34] Nobler MS, Sackeim HA, Louie J, et al. Clinical response to antidepressants is associated with reduced frontal CBF in late-life depression [abstract no. NR372. 1998]. Program and Abstracts on New Research. Presented at the one hundred fifty-first annual meeting of the American Psychiatric Association. Toronto, Ontario, Canada, May 30–June 4, 1998.
[35] Brody AL, Saxena S, Silverman DH, et al. Brain metabolic changes in major depressive disorder from pre- to post-treatment with paroxetine. Psychiatry Res 1999;91:127–39.
[36] Brody AL, Saxena S, Stoessel P, et al. Regional brain metabolic changes in patients with major depression treated with either paroxetine or interpersonal therapy: preliminary findings. Arch Gen Psychiatry 2001;58:631–40.
[37] Saletu B, Grunberger J, Linzmayer L, et al. The pharmacokinetics of nomifensine. Comparison of pharmacokinetics and pharmacodynamics using computer pharmaco-EEG. Int Pharmacopsychiatry 1982;17(Suppl 1):43–72.
[38] Saletu B, Grunberger J, Rajna P. Pharmaco-EEG profiles of antidepressants. Pharmacodynamic studies with fluvoxamine. Br J Clin Pharmacol 1983;15(Suppl 3):369S–83S.
[39] Saletu B, Grunberger J, Linzmayer L. On central effects of serotonin re-uptake inhibitors: quantitative EEG and psychometric studies with sertraline and zimelidine. J Neural Transm 1986;67(3–4):241–66.
[40] Saletu B, Anderer P, Kinsperger K, et al. Topographic brain mapping of EEG in neuropsychopharmacology–part II. Clinical applications (pharmaco EEG imaging). Methods Find Exp Clin Pharmacol 1987;9(6):385–408.
[41] Saletu B, Grunberger J. Classification and determination of cerebral bioavailability of fluoxetine: pharmacokinetic, pharmaco-EEG, and psychometric analyses. J Clin Psychiatry 1985;46(3 Pt 2):45–52.
[42] Saletu B, Grunberger J. Drug profiling by computed electroencephalography and brain maps, with special consideration of sertraline and its psychometric effects. J Clin Psychiatry 1988;49(Suppl):59–71.
[43] Sannita WG, Ottonello D, Perria B, et al. Topographic approaches in human quantitative pharmaco-electroencephalography. Neuropsychobiology 1983;9(1):66–72.
[44] Sannita WG. Quantitative EEG in human neuropharmacology. Rationale, history, and recent developments. Acta Neurol (Napoli) 1990;12(5):389–409.
[45] Itil TM, Menon GN, Bozak MM, et al. CNS effects of citalopram, a new serotonin inhibitor antidepressant (a quantitative pharmaco electroencephalography study). Prog Neuropsychopharmacol Biol Psychiatry 1984;8(3):397–409.
[46] Herrmann WM, Scharer E, Wendt G, et al. Pharmaco-EEG profile of levoprotiline: second example to discuss the predictive value of pharmaco-electroencephalography in early human pharmacological evaluations of psychoactive drugs. Pharmacopsychiatry 1991; 24(6):206–13.
[47] Luthringer R, Dago KT, Patat A, et al. Pharmacoelectroencephalographic profile of befloxatone, a new reversible MAO-A inhibitor, in healthy subjects. Neuropsychobiology 1996;34(2):98–105.
[48] Itil TM. The discovery of antidepressant drugs by computer-analyzed human cerebral bio-electrical potentials (CEEG). Prog Neurobiol 1983;20(3–4):185–249.
[49] Ulrich G, Renfordt E, Zeller G, et al. Interrelation between changes in the EEG and psychopathology under pharmacotherapy for endogenous depression. A contribution to the predictor question. Pharmacopsychiatry 1984;17(6):178–83.
[50] Ulrich G, Renfordt E, Frick K. The topographical distribution of alpha-activity in the resting EEG of endogenous-depressive in-patients with and without clinical response to pharmacotherapy. Pharmacopsychiatria 1986;19:272–3.

[51] Ulrich G, Renfordt E, Frick K. Electroencephalographic dynamics of vigilance and drug-response in endogenous depression. Pharmacopsychiatria 1986;19:270–1.

[52] Ulrich G, Haug HJ, Stieglitz RD, et al. EEG characteristics of clinically defined on-drug-responders and non-responders—a comparison clomipramine vs. maprotiline. Pharmacopsychiatry 1988;21(6):367–8.

[53] Ulrich G, Frick K. A new quantitative approach to the assessment of stages of vigilance as defined by spatiotemporal EEG patterning. Percept Mot Skills 1986;62(2):567–76.

[54] Knott VJ, Telner JI, Lapierre YD, et al. Quantitative EEG in the prediction of antidepressant response to imipramine. J Affect Disord 1996;39(3):175–84.

[55] Knott V, Mahoney C, Kennedy S, et al. Pre-treatment EEG and its relationship to depression severity and paroxetine treatment outcome. Pharmacopsychiatry 2000; 33(6):201–5.

[56] Saxena S, Brody AL, Ho ML, et al. Differential brain metabolic predictors of response to paroxetine in obsessive-compulsive disorder versus major depression. Am J Psychiatry 2003;160:522–32.

[57] Drevets WC, Bogers W, Raichle ME. Functional anatomical correlates of antidepressant drug treatment assessed using PET measures of regional glucose metabolism. Eur Neuropsychopharmacol 2002;12(6):527–44.

[58] Videbech P, Ravnkilde B, Pedersen TH, et al. The Danish PET/depression project: clinical symptoms and cerebral blood flow. A regions-of-interest analysis. Acta Psychiatr Scand 2002;106(1):35–44.

[59] Baxter LR Jr, Phelps ME, Mazziotta JC, et al. Local cerebral glucose metabolic rates in obsessive-compulsive disorder. A comparison with rates in unipolar depression and in normal controls. Arch Gen Psychiatry 1987;44(3):211–8.

[60] Drevets WC, Videen TO, Price JL, et al. A functional anatomical study of unipolar depression. J Neurosci 1992;12(9):3628–41.

[61] Bench CJ, Friston KJ, Brown RG, et al. The anatomy of melancholia—focal abnormalities of cerebral blood flow in major depression. Psychol Med 1992;22(3):607–15.

[62] Phan KL, Wager T, Taylor SF, et al. Functional neuroanatomy of emotion: a meta-analysis of emotion activation studies in PET and fMRI. Neuroimage 2002;16(2):331–48.

[63] Pizzagalli D, Pascual-Marqui RD, Nitschke JB, et al. Anterior cingulate activity as a predictor of degree of treatment response in major depression: evidence from brain electrical tomography analysis. Am J Psychiatry 2001;158(3):405–15.

[64] Pizzagalli DA, Oakes TR, Davidson RJ. Coupling of theta activity and glucose metabolism in the human rostral anterior cingulate cortex: an EEG/PET study of normal and depressed subjects. Psychophysiology 2003;40(6):939–49.

[65] Pizzagalli DA, Peccoralo LA, Davidson RJ, et al. Resting anterior cingulate activity and abnormal responses to errors in subjects with elevated depressive symptoms: a 128-channel EEG study. Hum Brain Mapp 2005; [Jul 20, Epub ahead of print].

[66] Davidson RJ, Henriques JB. Regional brain function in sadness and depression. In: Borod J, editor. The neuropsychology of emotion. New York: Oxford Univ Pres; 2000. p. 269–97.

[67] Henriques JB, Davidson RJ. Regional brain electrical asymmetries discriminate between previously depressed and healthy control subjects. J Abnorm Psychol 1990;99(1):22–31.

[68] Davidson RJ, Irwin W. The functional neuroanatomy of emotion and affective style. Trends Cogn Sci 1999;3(1):11–21.

[69] Davidson RJ. Anterior cerebral asymmetry and the nature of emotion. Brain Cogn 1992;20(1):125–51.

[70] Davidson RJ, Irwin W, Anderle MJ, et al. The neural substrates of affective processing in depressed patients treated with venlafaxine. Am J Psychiatry 2003;160(1):64–75.

[71] Bush G, Vogt BA, Holmes J, et al. Dorsal anterior cingulate cortex: a role in reward-based decision making. Proc Natl Acad Sci U S A 2002;99(1):523–8.

[72] Desiraju T. Electrophysiology of the frontal granular cortex. III. The cingulate-prefrontal relation in primate. Brain Res 1976;109(3):473–85.

[73] Vogt BA, Pandya DN. Cingulate cortex of the rhesus monkey: II. Cortical afferents. J Comp Neurol 1987;262(2):271–89.

[74] Koski L, Paus T. Functional connectivity of the anterior cingulate cortex within the human frontal lobe: a brain-mapping meta-analysis. Exp Brain Res 2000;133:55–65.

[75] Kumar A, Cook IA. White matter injury, neural connectivity and the pathophysiology of psychiatric disorders. Dev Neurosci 2002;24:255–61.

[76] Davidson RJ. Seven sins in the study of emotion: correctives from affective neuroscience. Brain Cogn 2003;52(1):129–32.

[77] Ishii R, Shinosaki K, Ukai S, et al. Medial prefrontal cortex generates frontal midline theta rhythm. Neuroreport 1999;10(4):675–9.

[78] Asada H, Fukuda Y, Tsunoda S, et al. Frontal midline theta rhythms reflect alternative activation of prefrontal cortex and anterior cingulate cortex in humans. Neurosci Lett 1999;274(1):29–32.

[79] Vinogradova OS. Expression, control, and probable functional significance of the neuronal theta-rhythm. Prog Neurobiol 1995;45:523–83.

[80] Basar E, Schurmann M, Sakowitz O. The selectively distributed theta system: functions. Int J Psychophysiol 2001;39(2–3):197–212.

[81] Aftanas LI, Golocheikine SA. Human anterior and frontal midline theta and lower alpha reflect emotionally positive state and internalized attention: high-resolution EEG investigation of meditation. Neurosci Lett 2001;310(1):57–60.

[82] Aftanas LI, Golocheikine SA. Non-linear dynamic complexity of the human EEG during meditation. Neurosci Lett 2002;330(2):143–6.

[83] Aftanas LI, Varlamov AA, Reva NV, et al. Disruption of early event-related theta synchronization of human EEG in alexithymics viewing affective pictures. Neurosci Lett 2003;340(1):57–60.

[84] Kubota Y, Sato W, Toichi M, et al. Frontal midline theta rhythm is correlated with cardiac autonomic activities during the performance of an attention demanding meditation procedure. Brain Res Cogn Brain Res 2001;11(2):281–7.

[85] Anderer P, Saletu B, Pascual-Marqui RD. Effect of the 5-HT(1A) partial agonist buspirone on regional brain electrical activity in man: a functional neuroimaging study using low-resolution electromagnetic tomography (LORETA). Psychiatry Res 2000;100(2):81–96.

[86] Knott VJ, Lapierre YD. Computerized EEG correlates of depression and antidepressant treatment. Prog Neuropsychopharmacol Biol Psychiatry 1987;11(2–3):213–21.

[87] Knott V, Mahoney C, Kennedy S, et al. EEG power, frequency, asymmetry and coherence in male depression. Psychiatry Res 2001;106(2):123–40.

[88] Knott V, Mahoney C, Kennedy S, et al. EEG correlates of acute and chronic paroxetine treatment in depression. J Affect Disord 2002;69(1–3):241–9.

[89] Heikman P, Salmelin R, Makela JP, et al. Relation between frontal 3-7 Hz MEG activity and the efficacy of ECT in major depression. J ECT 2001;17(2):136–40.

[90] Stubbeman WF, Leuchter AF, Cook IA, et al. Pretreatment neurophysiologic function and ECT response in depression. J ECT 2004;20(3):142–4.

[91] Iosifescu D, Greenwald SD, Devlin P, et al. Frontal EEG predicts clinical response to SSRI treatment in MDD [abstract #170]. Presented at the 44th annual meeting of the New Clinical Drug Evaluation Unit. Phoenix, AZ; June 1–4. 2004.

[92] Iosifescu DV, Greenwald S, Devlin P, et al. Pretreatment frontal EEG predicts changes in suicidal ideation during SSRI treatment in MDD. Presented at the 45th annual meeting of the New Clinical Drug Evaluation Unit (NCDEU). Boca Raton, FL; June 6–9, 2005.

[93] Iosifescu DV, Nierenberg AA, Mischoulon D, et al. An open study of triiodothyronine augmentation of selective serotonin reuptake inhibitors in treatment resistant major depressive disorder. J Clin Psychiatry 2005;66:1038–42.

[94] Poland R, Greenwald SD, Devlin P, et al. Change in frontal EEG predicts response to citalopram treatment in MDD [abstract #541]. Presented at the annual meeting of the American Psychiatric Association. Atlanta, GA; May 21–26, 2005.

[95] Leuchter AF, Cook IA, Lufkin RB, et al. Cordance: a new method for assessment of cerebral perfusion and metabolism using quantitative electroencephalography. Neuroimage 1994;1(3):208–19.

[96] Buchsbaum MS, Hazlett E, Sicotte N, et al. Geometric and scaling issues in topographic electroencephalography. In: Duffy FH, editor. Topographic mapping of brain electrical activity. Stoneham (MA): Butterworth Publishers; 1986. p. 325–37.

[97] Nagata K. Topographic EEG mapping in cerebrovascular disease. Brain Topogr 1989;2: 119–28.

[98] Wszolek ZK, Herkes GK, Lagerlund TD, et al. Comparison of EEG background frequency analysis, psychologic test scores, short tests of mental status, and quantitative SPECT in dementia. J Geriatr Psychiatry Neurol 1992;5:22–30.

[99] Leuchter AF, Cook IA, Newton TF, et al. Regional differences in brain electrical activity in dementia: use of spectral power and spectral ratio measures. Electroencephalogr Clin Neurophysiol 1993;87(6):385–93.

[100] Cook IA, Leuchter AF, Uijtdehaage SH, et al. Altered cerebral energy utilization in late life depression. J Affect Disord 1998;49(2):89–99.

[101] Leuchter AF, Uijtdehaage SH, Cook IA, et al. Relationship between brain electrical activity and cortical perfusion in normal subjects. Psychiatry Res 1999;90:125–40.

[102] Leuchter AF, Cook IA, Mena I, et al. Assessing cerebral perfusion using quantitative EEG cordance. Psych Res Neuroimaging 1994;55:141–52.

[103] Sackeim HA, Prohovnik I, Moeller JR, et al. Regional cerebral blood flow in mood disorders, I: comparison of major depressives and normal controls at rest. Arch Gen Psychiatry 1990;47:60–70.

[104] Cook I, Leuchter A. Prefrontal changes and treatment response prediction in depression. Semin Clin Neuropsychiatry 2001;6(2):113–20.

[105] Cook I, Leuchter A, Morgan M, et al. Early changes in prefrontal activity characterize clinical responders to antidepressants. Neuropsychopharmacology 2002;27(1): 120–31.

[106] Leuchter A, Cook I, Witte E, et al. Changes in brain function of depressed subjects during treatment with placebo. Am J Psychiatry 2002;159(1):122–9.

[107] Cook I, Leuchter A, Morgan M, et al. Changes in prefrontal activity characterize clinical response in SSRI nonresponders: a pilot study. J Psychiatr Res 2005;39(5):461–6.

[108] Bares M, Brunovsky M, Kopecek M, et al. Changes in QEEG prefrontal activity as a predictor of response to antidepressive medication in patients with treatment resistant depressive disorder: a pilot study. Presented at the 14th European Congress of Psychiatry, AEP. Nice, France, March 4–8, 2006.

[109] Kopecek M, Bares M, Brunovsky M, et al. EEG cordance as a predictor of response to antidepressive medication—pooled analysis. Presented at the 14th European Congress of Psychiatry, AEP. Nice, March 4–8, 2006.

[110] Leuchter AF, Cook IA, Hunter AM, et al. Functional brain changes associated with remission in major depressive disorder. Poster Presented at the meeting of the Society of Biological Psychiatry. Atlanta, GA; May 19–21, 2005.

[111] Cook IA, Hunter AM, Abrams M, et al. Midline and right frontal brain function and remission in major depression. Poster Presented at the 46th annual meeting of the New Clinical Drug Evaluation Unit (NCDEU). June 12–15, 2006.

[112] Hunter AM, Leuchter AF, Morgan ML, et al. Neurophysiologic correlates of side effects in normal subjects randomized to venlafaxine or placebo. Neuropsychopharmacology 2005;30(4):792–9.

[113] Scherg M, von Cramon D. Two bilateral sources of the late AEP as identified by a spatio-temporal dipole model. Electroencephalogr Clin Neurophysiol 1985;62:32–44.

[114] Paige SR, Fitzpatrik DF, Kline JP, et al. Event-related potential (ERP) amplitude/intensity slopes predict response to antidepressants. Neuropsychobiology 1994;30: 197–201.

[115] Lee TW, Yu YW, Chen TJ, et al. Loudness dependence of the auditory evoked potential and response to antidepressants in Chinese patients with major depression. J Psychiatry Neurosci 2005;30:202–5.
[116] Hegerl U, Juckel G. Intensity dependence of auditory evoked potentials as indicator of central serotonergic neurotransmission—a new hypothesis. Biol Psychiatry 1993;33:173–87.
[117] Gallinat J, Bottlender R, Juckel G, et al. The loudness dependency of the auditory evoked N1/P2 component as a predictor of the acute SSRI response in depression. Psychopharmacology 2000;148:404–11.
[118] Hegerl U, Herrmann WM. Event-related potentials and the prediction of differential drug response in psychiatry. Neuropsychobiology 1990;23:99–108.
[119] Linka T, Muller BW, Bender S, et al. The intensity dependence of the auditory evoked N1 component as a predictor of response to citalopram treatment in patients with major depression. Neurosci Lett 2004;367:375–8.
[120] Linka T, Muller BW, Bender S, et al. The intensity dependence of auditory evoked ERP components 123. Predicts responsiveness to reboxetine treatment in major depression. Pharmacopsychiatry 2005;38:139–43.
[121] Shils JL, Litt M, Skolnick BE, et al. Bispectral analysis of visual interactions in humans. Electroencephalogr Clin Neurophysiol 1996;98:113–25.
[122] Cook IA, Leuchter AF, Greenwald SD, et al. Single-channel EEG bispectrum predicts antidepressant treatment response. Poster Presented at the 42nd annual meeting of the New Clinical Drug Evaluation Unit Annual Meeting. Boca Raton, FL; May 28–31, 2002.

Psychiatr Clin N Am 30 (2007) 125–138

PSYCHIATRIC CLINICS
OF NORTH AMERICA

Pharmacogenetic Studies of Antidepressant Response: How Far from the Clinic?

Roy H. Perlis, MD, MSc

Pharmacogenetics Research Unit, Depression and Bipolar Clinical and Research Programs
and Center for Human Genetics Research, Massachusetts General Hospital, 15 Parkman St.,
WACC 812, Boston, MA 02114, USA

B oth the popular and the scientific press have embraced the idea of personalized medicine, in which genetic testing will allow precise matching of patients with optimal treatment [1–5]. Pharmacogenetics, the study of the way in which genetic variation influences response to drug treatment, may allow the further identification of novel drug targets and facilitate the development of entirely new interventions. In major depressive disorder, many patients fail to respond to, or to tolerate, an initial antidepressant trial [6–8]. Pharmacogenetic testing might provide an opportunity to decrease the number of treatment trials required to find an effective and well-tolerated treatment for a given patient and thus decrease the time during which the patient remains at risk for functional impairment and even suicide. To use pharmacogenetic testing effectively, clinicians will need to have a basic understanding of how such tests are developed and what their limitations are. The first portion of this article briefly defines basic concepts in pharmacogenetics as they pertain to psychiatry and then discusses their potential application in antidepressant pharmacogenetics. The second portion of the article addresses key obstacles to the development and application of such tests, so that clinicians can understand how to evaluate and apply new tests as they are developed.

PHARMACOGENETICS IN PSYCHIATRY

Early twin studies suggested that variation in the metabolism of a number of common drugs, among them tricyclic antidepressants, is heritable [9–11]. That is, if one twin was less able to metabolize a particular drug than the general population, the other twin also was likely to fall into this "poor metabolizer" category. In general, subsequent studies have suggested that only small subset of pharmacotherapies might be influenced by one or a few genes, whereas others are likely to be polygenic [12].

E-mail address: rperlis@partners.org

0193-953X/07/$ – see front matter
doi:10.1016/j.psc.2006.12.004

For psychotropic agents, and particularly antidepressants, the question of heritability is largely unstudied. Clinicians sometimes do make treatment decisions based on reports that a family member responded to a particular medication, for example, initiating treatment with a selective serotonin reuptake inhibitor (SSRI) because a sibling reportedly responded well to the same treatment. Although there is no reason to think antidepressant response is any less heritable than response to other pharmacotherapies, it is important to recognize that this hypothesis is less well supported than most other genetic-association studies in psychiatry (ie, it is much clearer that disorders such as major depressive disorder (MDD) or bipolar disorder are heritable).

Most pharmacogenetic studies investigate genes related to two processes involved in the actions of a drug. Pharmacokinetics describes the way in which a drug is distributed in or cleared from the body and involves absorption of the drug, distribution through hydrophilic and hydrophobic spaces, metabolism, and excretion. Of these processes, genes related to metabolism have received the most attention. Pharmacodynamics examines the drug's interaction with its receptors and transporters and with downstream processes such as second-messenger systems [13,14].

To understand the process of pharmacogenetics research, the example of the cytochrome p450 gene *CYP2D6* is instructive. Long before the gene was identified, it was known that individuals generally fall into one of four categories in their metabolic status for *CYP2D6*: poor, intermediate, wild-type (sometimes referred to as "extensive"), and ultra-rapid. The gene itself is quite small (4 kb); it lies on chromosome 22 and exhibits more than 50 different variations, primarily differences in numbers of copies of the gene. That is, some individuals have a deletion of this gene; others can have multiple copies. Many of these changes influence the amount of this enzyme produced and thus an individual's ability to metabolize the wide range of drugs that are affected by the 2D6 pathway [15]. Because variation is so common and affects so many drugs, this gene has been the basis of extensive study and early speculation that testing for this variation could affect clinical outcomes substantially, particularly in terms of adverse effects [16].

Beyond the potential benefits in personalizing treatment, the benefit of pharmacogenetics in identifying novel classes of pharmacotherapies also should be apparent. In the same way that finding genes associated with Alzheimer's disease helped open entirely new areas for drug development [17,18], identifying an unexpected gene or pathway involved in antidepressant efficacy could lead to novel treatment strategies in MDD.

A related concept is the idea of developing treatments for population subgroups, sometimes referred to as "minibusters" to distinguish them from the traditional drug development goal of "blockbusters" [12,19]. The US Food and Drug Administration (FDA) approval of the combination of isosorbide dinitrate/hydralazine hydrochloride specifically for individuals who identify themselves as black represented a first tentative step in this direction [20,21]. Other drugs that similarly failed to show benefit in large-scale studies but benefited particular genetic subgroups could be developed for niche populations once the genetic characteristics of such good responders are described [3].

Finally, pharmacogenetics may allow a faster drug-development process, culminating in drugs coming to market more quickly. Knowledge of genetic predictors might impact study design at several levels. If individuals at greater risk for study discontinuation because of adverse effects can be identified early in the process (ie, in phase II trials), they might be screened for and excluded from phase III trials, allowing smaller (and thus less expensive) studies with higher completion rates [22]. Likewise, if genes are found to be predictive of nonspecific (ie, placebo) response, it might be possible to exclude placebo responders and show greater differences between active drug and placebo or simply to study smaller cohorts to establish statistically significant differences.

BARRIERS TO APPLICATION

Despite the promise of pharmacogenetics, a number of significant obstacles continue to complicate the interpretation of such studies. Most of these barriers can be surmounted by collecting larger patient cohorts and using more sophisticated analytic approaches; some, however, will require greater attention early in study design to the potential application of the results. Ultimately, rather than simply being piggy-backed on existing clinical trials, clinical pharmacogenetics may require individual trials aimed at validating a specific test in a specific context. The following section highlights some of the barriers to progress in pharmacogenetics with a focus on their relevance in the pharmacogenetics of antidepressant response.

Need for Replication

As important as the *CYP2D6* gene has been in pharmacokinetics, the gene that codes the serotonin transporter has been equally crucial in the psychiatric study of pharmacodynamics. The serotonin transporter (5-hydroxytryptamine transporter [5HTT]) is the site of action of SSRIs and thus is a likely site at which variation might influence treatment response. Indeed, there is a common variation in the promoter region of this gene, in which a short stretch of DNA (44 base-pairs) is either present or absent; this region is referred to as the "5HTTLPR." It results in either a "short" or "long" form of the gene; the longer form has been associated with greater expression of 5HTT [23]. (Of note, more recent studies suggest that the 5HTTLPR may actually be triallelic; that is, a single-nucleotide polymorphism in this region also influences expression and may account for variable results in other 5HTT-association studies in psychiatry [24–26]).

Variation in the *5HTT* gene has been extensively studied in psychiatry, with associations reported to many disease states, particularly in mood and anxiety disorders, suggesting either a systematic source of type I error or that the gene may act as a vulnerability factor. Perhaps most notably, the 5HTTLPR polymorphism was associated with risk of developing MDD following stressful life events [27].

The 5HTTLPR also has been studied in numerous antidepressant treatment studies. One meta-analysis of 11 studies of this polymorphism in antidepressant treatment, which included primarily SSRIs but also included an investigation of sleep deprivation [28], suggested an association with treatment response [29]. In general, the long allele has been associated with better treatment response, or in some cases with more rapid antidepressant response, particularly in white cohorts [30,31]. Unfortunately, despite the apparent convergence of results, in the largest study to date, which was equivalent in size to all of the previous trials taken together and which used a rigorous prospective methodology, no evidence of association was detected [32]. Thus, the most recent evidence suggests that the best candidate association in antidepressant response does not replicate.

A similar story has emerged with the tryptophan hydroxylase enzyme, a key element of serotonin synthesis. The initial identification of a second form of this enzyme, TPH2, specifically expressed in brain, was reported with much fanfare [33], and a variation in TPH2 was associated with treatment resistance in a small number of patients [34]. Once again, however, when examined in a very large patient cohort, no evidence of association was detected [35].

This pattern—initial reports of association in small cohorts, followed by larger studies that see smaller associations or fail to confirm the association entirely—remains the norm in psychiatric genetics, and indeed in the genetics of complex diseases in general [36]. The most common explanation given is publication bias—that is, results that detect or confirm an initial association are more easily published than those that do not, so that only positive studies are disseminated. A related problem is that of multiple comparisons: it is common to see papers that report tests of multiple variations in multiple genes examining multiple phenotypes. In antidepressant pharmacogenetics, these reports often examine remission rates, changes in symptom severity, changes in symptom factors (eg, anxiety or core depression features), and time-to-onset. As the number of tests increases, the likelihood of identifying spurious associations increases as well. Lastl some reported associations may be the result of population stratification or admixture, discussed later.

Apparent Racial Differences

How informative, if at all, race and ethnicity are in genetic studies continues to generate heated debate [37]. As noted previously, evidence of racial differences in treatment response recently led to the approval of one drug combination for the treatment of hypertension in only self-identified blacks. Allele frequencies vary among racial groups, as the International Haplotype Map Project has demonstrated [38]. On the other hand, in general, self-identified race corresponds poorly to genetic variation.

One area in which race plays a potential role is its contribution to spurious associations. It has been suggested that antidepressant response differs among ethnic groups; however, this difference may be confounded (eg, by socioeconomic status). Allele frequencies, as noted previously, also vary across ethnic groups [38]. In such circumstances, population stratification is a concern in case-control studies: if allele frequencies differ by race, and race (either directly or as a proxy) is associated with differential outcome, the alleles may seem to be associated with differential outcome.

In psychiatric pharmacogenetics, a further difficulty has arisen in interpreting variation in the serotonin transporter promoter region. Most antidepressant studies in whites suggest that carrying at least one copy of the short allele confers a greater risk of antidepressant nonresponse, intolerance, or slower response [39]. On the other hand, in Southeast Asian populations, particularly Koreans and Japanese, the long allele seems to be the one associated with poorer or slower SSRI response [40,41]. If these effects are indeed real, it remains to be determined why the direction of association is opposite in different ethnic groups. It is counterintuitive that the same genetic variants would produce different effects in different populations if the variants are important determinants of drug response [30].

The variation in allele frequencies across racial groups also raises the possibility that a future gene-based diagnostic test may be informative only in one group or may be more informative in a particular group. For the cytochrome *P450 2D6* gene, for example, because the prior probability of carrying a variation associated with poor metabolism is much lower among nonwhites, the usefulness of testing could be lower for these groups. Indeed, the variation in populations is daunting: for three variants in *2D6* that cause poor metabolism, one (*P450 2D6*4*) is found largely in people of European ancestry, another (*2D6*17*) is found only in Africans, and *P450 2D6*10* is found in 70% of East Asians but is rare elsewhere. The ultra-rapid metabolizer phenotype was reported in about 5% of Spanish individuals but in 20% to 30% of Arab and Ethiopian individuals [13]. The same wide variation is seen in another p450 gene important in drug metabolism, *CYP2C19* [42]. Likewise, in a recent report by McMahon and colleagues [43], a variation in the 5HT$_{2A}$ receptor was associated significantly with response in whites but not in African-Americans, so a future test probably would need to incorporate additional markers to be informative in the latter group.

More broadly, because most cohorts used in pharmacogenetic studies are relatively small to begin with and focus on the largest group (typically whites) to minimize the potential for admixture, the possibility grows that some racial groups will be left out. The systematic collection of antidepressant response cohorts from nonwhite populations [44] may be required to obtain adequate information to estimate the performance of genetic tests in these groups.

Recently the debate about reporting clinical trial results according to race has become more prominent, but no consensus has yet emerged [45–47]. Ultimately pharmacogenetic testing should become sophisticated enough that self-identified race will not be particularly useful; in the near-term, however, it may be needed to determine which populations are likely to benefit more from a given set of tests [47–50].

Need for Active Comparator Studies

A crucial but often overlooked feature of clinically informative pharmacogenetic studies is the presence of an active comparator. Most pharmacogenetic studies to date have examined overall treatment response to a single agent. Without a comparator drug, the specificity of association cannot be established: for example, particular genes might be associated with poorer treatment response regardless of modality. This sort of test still might allow a clinician to prioritize patients according to risk of nonresponse. Those at higher risk for nonresponse might receive earlier augmentation, more frequent visits, or the addition of a structured psychotherapy. Still, in general, knowing that an individual is less likely to respond to treatment is much less useful than knowing that an individual is more likely to respond to another treatment.

Two examples are informative. The first is an examination of paroxetine and mirtazapine in geriatric depression, Murphy and colleagues [51] found greater discontinuation among individuals who had a polymorphism in the $5HT_{2A}$ receptor treated with paroxetine but not with mirtazapine. (Overall response rates did not differ between the two groups). Armed with this sort of test, a clinician might elect to initiate treatment with mirtazapine preferentially in patients at high risk for discontinuation.

A second comparator study examined a cohort of Korean patients who had late-life depression treated with fluoxetine, sertraline, or the norepinephrine reuptake inhibitor (NRI) nortriptyline [52]. Notably, although the serotonin transporter was associated with differential response to either the serotonin reuptake inhibitor (SRI) or NRI, a polymorphism in the norepinephrine transporter was associated with greater NRI but not SRI response. Among those individuals homozygous for the G allele of the NET G1287A single-nucleotide polymorphism, the response rate to NRI was 83.3%, compared with 58.7% for SRI. Although tricyclic antidepressant agents generally are relegated to second- or third-line treatment today because of the availability of safer agents, the risk–benefit relationship might change in individuals who have this particular genotype, with NRI favored as first-line again.

Need to Consider Adverse Effects

Most pharmacogenomic studies have focused on antidepressant efficacy rather than on aspects of tolerability, probably because efficacy typically is the primary endpoint in the clinical trials from which these cohorts derived. Adverse effects also are generally more rare than endpoints such as response (ie, a 50% decrease in symptoms at endpoint), which limits power to detect effects in association studies. Finally, as with efficacy, the assumption that adverse-effect liability is familial is rarely tested directly; one notable exception was a small twin study suggesting the plateau weight with clozapine treatment is heritable [53].

On the other hand, adverse effects offer three substantial advantages over other treatment-response phenotypes for genetic studies. First, they typically are measured more reliably: individuals either develop insomnia, or they do not. Second, they may be more treatment specific than clinical improvement: the incidence of many adverse effects differs markedly between antidepressants and placebo, but clinical improvement, unfortunately, does not. Third, in some cases the pathophysiology associated with adverse effects may be slightly clearer, offering better insight in the selection of candidate genes for study.

Adverse effects also have substantial clinical importance. Beyond their impact on quality of life, adverse effects frequently lead to medication discontinuation. In a primary care setting, adverse effects are the primary reason cited for noncompliance and discontinuation by patients treated with antidepressants [6,54], and 50% or more of patients terminate antidepressant treatment prematurely [55]. Indeed, noncompliance may be as high as 70% to 80% for patients who have psychotic disorders and 60% for outpatients who have MDD [56].

Among the most common adverse effects with SSRIs in particular are weight gain, insomnia, and sexual dysfunction. The author and colleagues were unable to identify any published analyses of SSRI-associated weight gain, possibly because few cohorts are followed long enough to see an effect. The pharmacogenetic literature for weight gain with antipsychotics is intriguing: one typical study of clozapine-treated patients (n = 117) found a variation in the $5HT_{2C}$ receptor to be associated with significantly less risk for weight gain [57], findings consistent with at least one subsequent study [58].

For insomnia, a preliminary report from the author's group suggested an association between the 5HTTLPR short allele and fluoxetine treatment–emergent insomnia as well as activating side effects, including akathisia. This finding was consistent with a number of studies in bipolar patients suggesting an association with antidepressant treatment–emergent mania.

Until recently, sexual dysfunction had been ignored in pharmacogenetic studies, despite its marked impact on adherence. A study of SSRI discontinuation indicated that sexual adverse effects were a primary or secondary reason for discontinuation in more than 30% of patients [59]. In a survey of patients, nearly 90% believed that antidepressant-associated sexual dysfunction warranted treatment discontinuation [60]. A recent report identified an association between a variation in the gene coding for the $5HT_{2A}$ receptor and SSRI-emergent sexual dysfunction; those who had two copies of a particular polymorphism were approximately 3.6 times more likely to experience sexual dysfunction, particularly relating to arousal [61]. Given the small sample size and consequent wide confidence interval, replication is necessary, but at a minimum studies like this indicate the potential role pharmacogenetics could play in addressing adverse effects.

Debate continues as to whether antidepressants cause some patients to develop increased suicidal thinking or behavior. It is clear, however, that a subset of patients who did not have suicidal thoughts before beginning antidepressant may develop such thoughts after antidepressant initiation. The prevalence of such a phenomenon varies depending on precise definition but seems to range from about 8% to 15% [62–64]. Two recent reports examined genetic predictors of treatment-associated suicidality. In the first, the author's group examined the *CREB1* gene, which previously had been associated with differential anger control among males [65]. Variations in *CREB* expression or phosphorylation also have been associated with suicide, particularly violent suicide, and in antidepressant effects in animal models. Among citalopram-treated patients drawn from the multicenter Sequenced Treatment Alternatives to Relieve Depression (STAR*D) study, the risk allele was associated with an approximately threefold increased risk of developing suicidal thinking, but only among males. Using a similar approach, McMahon and colleagues [66] recently have reported preliminary evidence of association for glutamatergic genes and treatment-emergent suicidal ideation.

Determining Test Parameters

A common problem in analyses that attempt to model a dependent variable as a function of independent predictors (for example, logistic regression) is over-fitting: the model performs well in the sample in which it was derived but much less well in other, noisier samples. This problem probably accounts for the rarity with which clinical predictors of outcome in mood disorders are replicated [67]. In a large clinical trials database, for example, the author and colleagues found certain predictors of a bipolar (versus MDD) diagnosis and reported classification accuracy of 87% [68]. Such predictions nearly always are optimistic, however, overestimating the model's performance in other data sets.

A crucial fact for nongeneticists to keep in mind is that a pharmacogenetic test is, in essence, no different from any other test used in medicine. As such, its value depends on the context in which it is used. A key first question is, "Will the results of this test change my management of the patient?" If not, the value of the test obviously is in question. Another important factor to consider for any test that does not have perfect sensitivity and specificity is the prior probability of whatever is being tested for. If the prior probability is low, the likelihood of a false-positive result goes up. On the other hand, in some circumstances, clinicians might be willing to accept a highly sensitive, even if somewhat nonspecific, test. One such circumstance would involve testing for rare but potentially serious adverse effects, such as Stevens-Johnson syndrome following lamotrigine treatment: the consequences of a false-negative result would far outweigh those of a false positive.

As with any other decision or intervention, pharmacogenetic tests can be evaluated using cost-effectiveness analyses, although this approach has been applied rarely to date. One study suggested cost effectiveness for a test of a common polymorphism that has been associated with toxicity from azathioprine, a drug used to treat autoimmune disease [69] The author's group recently applied cost-effectiveness analysis to examine a test for clozapine treatment response, one of the few to report sensitivity and specificity (although these findings must be interpreted with the caveats noted previously) [70,71]. Two strategies were compared—treating all patients who had schizophrenia with a typical neuroleptic first and reserving clozapine for the failures, or treating the likely responders with clozapine first. In this model, the test, even though its Bayesian parameters are only modest, performed well enough to yield cost savings over a range of conditions. The cost per quality-adjusted life year (QALY), a common measure of outcome, was nearly $50,000; by comparison, a quality-improvement program for antidepressant use in primary care was estimated to cost between $15,000 and $36,000 per QALY, and an examination of 587 lifesaving medical interventions yielded a median cost of $42,000 per QALY. Although the validity of the clozapine test itself has been questioned, and the clinical situation modeled is somewhat artificial, this approach can be applied to examine any new pharmacogenetic test. Indeed, the author's group has developed a similar model for antidepressant response based on results from the landmark STAR*D study in MDD (R. Perlis, A. Patrick, and P. Wang, unpublished data, 2007).

Determining Test Application

The first pharmacogenetic test to enter widespread clinical application examines common variations in two pharmacokinetic enzyme genes, *CYP450 2D6* and *2C19* [72]. These variations allow the classification of individuals into various categories by how well they metabolize particular groups of drugs, as discussed previously.

One limitation of such testing is that environmental factors also are known to influence drug metabolism. Perhaps the most common factor is other medications: cotreatment with a drug that inhibits *P450 2D6*, such as paroxetine, may make an individual who otherwise is genetically a wild-type or normal metabolizer seem to be a poor metabolizer. Other factors that may vary over time relate to diet, medical illness, and age. Therefore, knowing an individual's genetic predisposition provides only partial information about his or her metabolic status at any given time. Environmental exposures, which include anything from dyes to diet (eg, preservatives, Brussels sprouts, cabbage, charcoal-broiled beef, and grapefruit juice), can have a marked impact on metabolic status [73–76]. Another key environmental exposure for much of the general population is nicotine and caffeine [42,77]. Drinking one 8-oz glass of grapefruit juice can inhibit *P450 3A4* for up 2 days, with consequent increase in levels of lamotrigine, carbamazepine, tricyclic agents, and clozapine [78]. Similarly, concentrations of neuroleptics and antidepressants may be decreased by as much as half by cigarette smoking, and there are reports of drug toxicity following smoking cessation.

Indeed, in many cases simply checking the blood level of a particular drug is the easiest way to define metabolic status. Still, these difficulties can be addressed in part by gathering additional data about other medications, medical history, and diet.

For a test to be useful, however, it also is critical to know how it fits into a particular decision algorithm, that is, how will those who have a positive test be treated differently from those who have a negative test. For pharmacokinetic tests in particular, this determination entails detailed data about drug kinetics in various metabolic contexts: how does it behave in poor metabolizers

compared with wild-type compared with ultra-rapid metabolizers? Unfortunately, the package insert or the *Physician's Desk Reference* information for most
drugs shows that the data come from a limited number of individuals, usually
normal volunteers or those who have particular comorbidity (ie, hepatic
disease). Although this information may be useful for defining average drug
doses in the general population, it reveals little about optimal dosing in specific
subgroups.

A recent review of psychiatric pharmacogenetics shows a bar graph with
potential dosing adjustments by metabolic status for a variety of drugs [29]. Developing such an algorithm would be useful for incorporating pharmacokinetic
tests into practice. This figure, however, is based on very limited numbers of
patients and requires extrapolation from general assumptions about the impact
of metabolic status to effects on specific drugs.

SUMMARY

Because the US FDA has begun to focus on disclosure of pharmacogenetic testing results in applications for new drug approval and review of existing drugs
(see, eg, http://www.fda.gov/OHRMS/DOCKETS/AC/05/slides/2005-4194S1_
Slide-Index.htm), the application of such testing in a clinical setting is likely to
increase substantially. Instead of small cohorts of patients, potentially nearly every participant in the large pivotal trials required for drug approval could help
inform the future application of that drug. Psychiatry as a whole, and antidepressant prescribing in particular, stands to benefit in the near term from the
ability to match patients and treatments better and in the longer term from
the identification of newer treatment targets that may overcome some of the
limitations of current therapeutics. On the other hand, despite the excitement
about the rapid pace of development in psychiatric pharmacogenetics, a number
of key issues remain to be addressed before these discoveries are applied in
a clinical setting. Close coordination will be required between those who study
treatment efficacy and effectiveness and those who study genetic variation in
populations to ensure that studies yield results that have scientific importance
and clinical importance as well.

References

[1] Lai TJ, Wu CY, Tsai HW, et al. Polymorphism screening and haplotype analysis of the tryp-
    tophan hydroxylase gene (TPH1) and association with bipolar affective disorder in Taiwan.
    BMC Med Genet 2005;6:14.
[2] Kaplan A. Advances in pharmacogenomics reduce side effects and save lives. Psychiatric
    Times 2005;22(1):4–7.
[3] Koppal T. Designing personalized medicines. Drug Discovery & Development 2003
    April:30–34.
[4] Evans WE, McLeod HL. Pharmacogenomics—drug disposition, drug targets, and side ef-
    fects. N Engl J Med 2003;348(6):538–49.
[5] Evans WE, Relling MV. Pharmacogenomics: translating functional genomics into rational
    therapeutics. Science 1999;286(5439):487–91.
[6] Katon W, von Korff M, Lin E, et al. Adequacy and duration of antidepressant treatment in
    primary care. Med Care 1992;30(1):67–76.

[7] Rush AJ, Fava M, Wisniewski SR, et al. Sequenced treatment alternatives to relieve depression (STAR*D): rationale and design. Control Clin Trials 2004;(25):118–41.
[8] Fava M. Diagnosis and definition of treatment-resistant depression. Biol Psychiatry 2003; 53(8):649–59.
[9] Vesell ES, Page JG. Genetic control of drug levels in man: antipyrine. Science 1968; 161(836):72–3.
[10] Vesell ES, Page JG. Genetic control of drug levels in man: phenylbutazone. Science 1968;159(822):1479–80.
[11] Vesell ES. Intraspecies differences in frequency of genes directly affecting drug disposition: the individual factor in drug response. Pharmacol Rev 1978;30(4):555–63.
[12] Melzer D, Raven A, Detmer DE, et al. My very own medicine: what I must know: information policy for pharmacogenetics. Cambridge (MA): University of Cambridge; 2003.
[13] Lin KM, Smith MW, Ortiz V. Culture and psychopharmacology. Psychiatr Clin North Am 2001;24(3):523–38.
[14] Tate SK, Goldstein DB. Will tomorrow's medicines work for everyone? Nat Genet 2004;36(11 Suppl):S34–42.
[15] Kroemer HK, Eichelbaum M. "It's the genes, stupid". Molecular bases and clinical consequences of genetic cytochrome P450 2D6 polymorphism. Life Sci 1995;56(26):2285–98.
[16] Meyer UA. Pharmacogenetics and adverse drug reactions. Lancet 2000;356(9242): 1667–71.
[17] Tomita T, Iwatsubo T. The inhibition of gamma-secretase as a therapeutic approach to Alzheimer's disease. Drug News Perspect 2004;17(5):321–5.
[18] Espeseth AS, Xu M, Huang Q, et al. Compounds that bind APP and inhibit Abeta processing in vitro suggest a novel approach to Alzheimer disease therapeutics. J Biol Chem 2005; 280(18):17792–7.
[19] Roses AD. Reducing pipeline attrition in clinical development via pharmacogenetics. Drug Discovery & Development 2003 August:15.
[20] Taylor AL, Ziesche S, Yancy C, et al. Combination of isosorbide dinitrate and hydralazine in blacks with heart failure. N Engl J Med 2004;351(20):2049–57.
[21] Saul S. FDA approves a heart drug for African-Americans. New York Times. June 24, 2005, Section C2.
[22] Goldstein DB. Pharmacogenetics in the laboratory and the clinic. N Engl J Med 2003;348(6):553–6.
[23] Heils A, Teufel A, Petri S, et al. Allelic variation of human serotonin transporter gene expression. J Neurochem 1996;66(6):2621–4.
[24] Hu XZ, Lipsky RH, Zhu G, et al. Serotonin transporter promoter gain-of-function genotypes are linked to obsessive-compulsive disorder. Am J Hum Genet 2006;78(5):815–26.
[25] Parsey RV, Hastings RS, Oquendo MA, et al. Effect of a triallelic functional polymorphism of the serotonin-transporter-linked promoter region on expression of serotonin transporter in the human brain. Am J Psychiatry 2006;163(1):48–51.
[26] Zalsman G, Huang YY, Oquendo MA, et al. Association of a triallelic serotonin transporter gene promoter region (5-HTTLPR) polymorphism with stressful life events and severity of depression. Am J Psychiatry 2006;163(9):1588–93.
[27] Caspi A, Sugden K, Moffitt TE, et al. Influence of life stress on depression: moderation by a polymorphism in the 5-HTT gene. Science 2003;301(5631):386–9.
[28] Benedetti F, Serretti A, Colombo C, et al. Influence of a functional polymorphism within the promoter of the serotonin transporter gene on the effects of total sleep deprivation in bipolar depression. Am J Psychiatry 1999;156(9):1450–2.
[29] Kirchheiner J, Nickchen K, Bauer M, et al. Pharmacogenetics of antidepressants and antipsychotics: the contribution of allelic variations to the phenotype of drug response. Mol Psychiatry 2004;9(5):442–73.
[30] Mancama D, Kerwin RW. Role of pharmacogenomics in individualising treatment with SSRIs. CNS Drugs 2003;17(3):143–51.

[31] Zanardi R, Benedetti F, Di Bella D, et al. Efficacy of paroxetine in depression is influenced by a functional polymorphism within the promoter of the serotonin transporter gene. J Clin Psychopharmacol 2000;20(1):105–7.

[32] Kraft JB, Peters EJ, Slager SL, et al. Analysis of Association Between the Serotonin Transporter and Antidepressant Response in a Large Clinical Sample. Biol Psychiatry. 2006 Nov 20; [Epub ahead of print].

[33] Zhang X, Beaulieu JM, Sotnikova TD, et al. Tryptophan hydroxylase-2 controls brain serotonin synthesis. Science 2004;305(5681):217.

[34] Zill P, Baghai TC, Zwanzger P, et al. SNP and haplotype analysis of a novel tryptophan hydroxylase isoform (TPH2) gene provide evidence for association with major depression. Mol Psychiatry 2004;9(11):1030–6.

[35] Zhou Z, Peters EJ, Hamilton SP, et al. Response to Zhang et al. (2005): loss-of-function mutation in tryptophan hydroxylase-2 identified in unipolar major depression. Neuron 45, 11-16. Neuron 2005;48(5):702–3 [author reply: 705–6].

[36] Hirschhorn JN, Altshuler D. Once and again—issues surrounding replication in genetic association studies. J Clin Endocrinol Metab 2002;87(10):4438–41.

[37] Jones DS, Perlis RH. Pharmacogenetics, race, and psychiatry: prospects and challenges. Harv Rev Psychiatry 2006;14(2):92–108.

[38] Sachidanandam R, Weissman D, Schmidt SC, et al. A map of human genome sequence variation containing 1.42 million single nucleotide polymorphisms. Nature 2001;409(6822): 928–33.

[39] Serretti A, Cusin C, Rausch JL, et al. Pooling pharmacogenetic studies on the serotonin transporter: a mega-analysis. Psychiatry Res 2006;145(1):61–5.

[40] Kim DK, Lim SW, Lee S, et al. Serotonin transporter gene polymorphism and antidepressant response. Neuroreport 2000;11(1):215–9.

[41] Yoshida K, Ito K, Sato K, et al. Influence of the serotonin transporter gene-linked polymorphic region on the antidepressant response to fluvoxamine in Japanese depressed patients. Prog Neuropsychopharmacol Biol Psychiatry 2002;26(2):383–6.

[42] Bertilsson L. Geographical/interracial differences in polymorphic drug oxidation. Current state of knowledge of cytochromes P450 (CYP) 2D6 and 2C19. Clin Pharmacokinet 1995;29(3):192–209.

[43] McMahon FJ, Buervenich S, Charney D, et al. Variation in the gene encoding the serotonin 2A receptor is associated with outcome of antidepressant treatment. Am J Hum Genet 2006;78(5):804–14.

[44] Licinio J, O'Kirwan F, Irizarry K, et al. Association of a corticotropin-releasing hormone receptor 1 haplotype and antidepressant treatment response in Mexican-Americans. Mol Psychiatry 2004;9(12):1075–82.

[45] Cooper RS, Kaufman JS, Ward R. Race and genomics. N Engl J Med 2003;348(12): 1166–70.

[46] Burchard EG, Ziv E, Coyle N, et al. The importance of race and ethnic background in biomedical research and clinical practice. N Engl J Med 2003;348(12):1170–5.

[47] Phimister EG. Medicine and the racial divide. N Engl J Med 2003;348(12):1081–2.

[48] Wilson JF, Weale ME, Smith AC, et al. Population genetic structure of variable drug response. Nat Genet 2001;29(3):265–9.

[49] Bloche MG. Race-based therapeutics. N Engl J Med 2004;351(20):2035–7.

[50] Jorde LB, Wooding SP. Genetic variation, classification and 'race'. Nat Genet 2004;36(11 Suppl):S28–33.

[51] Murphy GM Jr, Hollander SB, Rodrigues HE, et al. Effects of the serotonin transporter gene promoter polymorphism on mirtazapine and paroxetine efficacy and adverse events in geriatric major depression. Arch Gen Psychiatry 2004;61(11):1163–9.

[52] Kim H, Lim SW, Kim S, et al. Monoamine transporter gene polymorphisms and antidepressant response in Koreans with late-life depression. JAMA 2006;296(13):1609–18.

[53] Theisen FM, Gebhardt S, Haberhausen M, et al. Clozapine-induced weight gain: a study in monozygotic twins and same-sex sib pairs. Psychiatr Genet 2005;15(4):285–9.

[54] Lin EH, Von Korff M, Katon W, et al. The role of the primary care physician in patients' adherence to antidepressant therapy. Med Care 1995;33(1):67–74.

[55] Melartin TK, Rytsala HJ, Leskela US, et al. Continuity is the main challenge in treating major depressive disorder in psychiatric care. J Clin Psychiatry 2005;66(2):220–7.

[56] Breen R, Thornhill JT. Noncompliance with medication for psychiatric disorders. CNS Drugs 1998;9:457–71.

[57] Reynolds GP, Zhang ZJ, Zhang XB. Association of antipsychotic drug-induced weight gain with a 5-HT2C receptor gene polymorphism. Lancet 2002;359(9323):2086–7.

[58] Reynolds GP, Zhang Z, Zhang X. Polymorphism of the promoter region of the serotonin 5-HT(2C) receptor gene and clozapine-induced weight gain. Am J Psychiatry 2003; 160(4):677–9.

[59] Bull SA, Hunkeler EM, Lee JY, et al. Discontinuing or switching selective serotonin-reuptake inhibitors. Ann Pharmacother 2002;36(4):578–84.

[60] Hirschfeld RM, Lewis L, Vornik LA. Perceptions and impact of bipolar disorder: how far have we really come? Results of the National Depressive and Manic-Depressive Association 2000 survey of individuals with bipolar disorder. J Clin Psychiatry 2003;64(2): 161–74.

[61] Bishop JR, Moline J, Ellingrod VL, et al. Serotonin 2A -1438 G/A and G-protein Beta3 sub-unit C825T polymorphisms in patients with depression and SSRI-associated sexual side-effects. Neuropsychopharmacology 2006;31(10):2281–8.

[62] Perlis RH, Beasley CM Jr, Wines JD Jr, et al. Treatment-associated suicidal ideation and adverse effects in an open, multicenter trial of fluoxetine for major depressive episodes. Psychother Psychosom 2007;76(1):40–6.

[63] Beasley CM, Disch D, Prabhakar V, et al. Potential Risk Factors for Development of Treat-ment-emergent Suicidal Ideation/Acts in the Fluoxetine Placebo-controlled Major Depres-sive Disorder Database. Presented at American College of Neuropsychopharmacology, Boca Raton, FL; 2006.

[64] Perlis RH, Purcell S, Fava M, et al. Association between treatment-emergent suicidal ideation with citalopram and polymorphisms near cAMP Response Element Binding Protein (CREB1) in the STAR*D study. Archives of General Psychiatry, in press.

[65] Perlis RH, Purcell S, Fagerness J, et al. Clinical and Genetic Dissection of Anger Expression and CREB1 Polymorphisms in Major Depressive Disorder. Biol Psych, in press.

[66] McMahon, et al. Abstract presented at the American Society of Human Genetics. 2006.

[67] Perlis RH, Iosifescu DV, Renshaw PF. Biological predictors of treatment response in affective illness. Psychiatr Clin North Am 2003;26(2):323–44.

[68] Perlis RH, Brown E, Baker RW, et al. Clinical features of bipolar depression versus major depressive disorder in large multicenter trials. Am J Psychiatry 2006;163(2):225–31.

[69] Marra CA, Esdaile JM, Anis AH. Practical pharmacogenetics: the cost effectiveness of screening for thiopurine s-methyltransferase polymorphisms in patients with rheumatologi-cal conditions treated with azathioprine. J Rheumatol 2002;29(12):2507–12.

[70] Arranz MJ, Munro J, Birkett J, et al. Pharmacogenetic prediction of clozapine response. Lancet 2000;355(9215):1615–6.

[71] Perlis RH, Ganz DA, Avorn J, et al. Pharmacogenetic testing in the clinical management of schizophrenia: a decision-analytic model. J Clin Psychopharmacol 2005;25(5):427–34.

[72] Anonymous web site: Amlichip CYP450 test. Available at: http://www.roche.com/ prod_diag_amplichip.htm.

[73] Pantuck EJ, Hsiao KC, Conney AH, et al. Effect of charcoal-broiled beef on phenacetin metabolism in man. Science 1976;194(4269):1055–7.

[74] Pantuck EJ, Kuntzman R, Conney AH. Decreased concentration of phenacetin in plasma of cigarette smokers. Science 1972;175(27):1248–50.

[75] Conney AH, Pantuck EJ, Hsiao KC, et al. Enhanced phenacetin metabolism in human subjects fed charcoal-broiled beef. Clin Pharmacol Ther 1976;20(6):633–42.

[76] Alvares AP, Pantuck EJ, Anderson KE, et al. Regulation of drug metabolism in man by environmental factors. Drug Metab Rev 1979;9(2):185–205.

[77] Lin KM, Poland RE, Anderson D. Psychopharmacology, ethnicity, and culture. Transcultural Psychiatric Research 1995;32:3–40.

[78] Wilkinson GR. Drug metabolism and variability among patients in drug response. N Engl J Med 2005;352(21):2211–21.

PSYCHIATRIC CLINICS
OF NORTH AMERICA

ELSEVIER
SAUNDERS

INDEX

Note: Page numbers of article titles are in **boldface** type.

0193-953X/07/$ – see front matter
doi:10.1016/S0193-953X(07)00026-3

Moving?

Make sure your subscription moves with you!

To notify us of your new address, find your **Clinics Account Number** (located on your mailing label above your name), and contact customer service at:

E-mail: elspcs@elsevier.com

800-654-2452 (subscribers in the U.S. & Canada)
407-345-4000 (subscribers outside of the U.S. & Canada)

Fax number: 407-363-9661

Elsevier Periodicals Customer Service
6277 Sea Harbor Drive
Orlando, FL 32887-4800

*To ensure uninterrupted delivery of your subscription, please notify us at least 4 weeks in advance of move.